RECONNECTING
to
SELF-HEALING

The Art of Advocating for Yourself

VALENTINA CASTRO

BALBOA.PRESS
A DIVISION OF HAY HOUSE

Balboa Press books may be ordered through booksellers or by contacting:

Balboa Press
A Division of Hay House
1663 Liberty Drive
Bloomington, IN 47403
www.balboapress.com
1 (877) 407-4847

Because of the dynamic nature of the Internet, any web addresses or links contained in this book may have changed since publication and may no longer be valid. The views expressed in this work are solely those of the author and do not necessarily reflect the views of the publisher, and the publisher hereby disclaims any responsibility for them.

The author of this book does not dispense medical advice or prescribe the use of any technique as a form of treatment for physical, emotional, or medical problems without the advice of a physician, either directly or indirectly. The intent of the author is only to offer information of a general nature to help you in your quest for emotional and spiritual well-being. In the event you use any of the information in this book for yourself, which is your constitutional right, the author and the publisher assume no responsibility for your actions.

Any people depicted in stock imagery provided by Getty Images are models, and such images are being used for illustrative purposes only. Certain stock imagery © Getty Images.

Painting by: Valentina Castro
Photo by: Hansel Solera

Print information available on the last page.

ISBN: 978-1-9822-3997-8 (sc)
ISBN: 978-1-9822-3998-5 (hc)
ISBN: 978-1-9822-3999-2 (e)

Library of Congress Control Number: 2019920678

Balboa Press rev. date: 12/12/2019

PRAISES

"Reconnecting to self-healing is treasure trove of information and guidance for those who are currently facing (or will face) major obstacles. Valentina beautifully shares how our greatest challenges can (and likely are created to) bring out the best in us. I am certain that this fresh perspective will empower many to both survive and thrive".
Robert A. Rakowski, DC, CCN, DACBN, DIBAK
Natural Medicine Center
Houston, TX

"In recent years there have been so many advances in medicine, particularly the treatment of lung cancer. Valentina in her journey, share with us the importance of her attitude as a powerful tool for healing. I know that this book will help people with cancer and many other diseases to never lose hope."
Dr. Jorge Alatorre Alexander
National Institute of Respiratory Diseases (INER)
Thoracic Oncology Clinic
Mexico City

"Valentina Castro has been a student of Truth in all the years that I have known her.
As she has met this physical challenge, I have admired her strength, courage, and determination to remain true to her own inner guidance from her own still small voice within, to heal her body. She has done so in spite of that appearance of truth that dominates our sense conscious world. When we rely on the human limitations of our current knowledge, we don't rely on the absolute Truth of the world of all possibilities that are innate in us all. When we combine science with our higher divine spirit and operate from that realm of true power we will be made whole. In

the philosophy of New Thought and the practice of metaphysics, we understand we are both human and divine and the divine of us is far more powerful than the limited of us. Valentina is that rare individual that embraces the whole of herself that is made up of both. She honors and relies on her whole being, and she will overcome all challenges because she will embrace them both. This journey her soul has chosen will be a beacon of light for healing and wholeness to all who follow her teachings".

Reverend Farolyn Mann
Senior Minister at Unity Church in Rockport, Tx

PREFACE

For perhaps fifteen years, I have had the desire to write a book. I have collaborated on magazine articles, and I am passionate about reading. I had the dream of writing a novel, but every time I sat down to begin, I realized I had nothing exciting to tell.

Now, life gives me the opportunity to have a story with a real message to share. Although my inner voice has told me, *Write a book*, since I received my diagnosis, almost every day I've written in my art journal. Since I began this journey, my inner voice has told me: *You have to write a book*. And that's how this book in your hands was born. This book is written from the heart and should be read from the heart as well. And it aims to guide the reader toward healing.

DISCLAIMER

In this book, I share healing techniques and suggestions that contribute to coping with the cancer process (and other disease). It is a complement to conventional and/or alternative methods that the reader elects for a cure. At no time is this book intended to replace any doctor or treatment, nor is it intended to diagnose.

The experiences I share are based on my own. The cases I present in chapter 8 are people with whom I have worked who have given me permission to share their stories. (For reasons of confidentiality, I have changed their names.)

Likewise, this book is not intended as a medical book but rather a scientific one. (There is scientific evidence of how our biology responds to events in our lives.) I have not described the complexity of neuroscience—that's not the goal of this book. The science I use is the science and wisdom of the nature of our bodies. For this, I relied on books I have read (see the reference section at the end of the book) and on my personal and professional experience.

I dedicate this book to you, my friend, that life has put you on your path. A mountain that suddenly seems difficult to climb is actually an opportunity to start a journey full of learning and the chance to deeply know yourself and to help you find your secret way for self-healing. You will see that the mountain was not that high after all.

I also dedicate this book to my beloved husband, Alberto, my life partner, my anchor, my best friend, my soul mate, and father of our four children—Santiago, Emilio, Tatiana, and Julia. They are my inspiration and my teachers; they have forced me to expand the limits of my beliefs, helped me to know and question myself and, above all, to become aware of the task of guiding them to be the best versions of themselves to contribute better human beings for this world.

I also dedicate this book to my parents, whom I honor for giving me life—my mother and stepfather, with their love, have done what is humanly possible in providing me with the tools for life—and to my brothers, for their presence in my life.

May we all keep together in our different life projects as individuals and as a family, always surrounded by unconditional love.

CONTENTS

FOREWORD

Dr. James Forsythe:

Valentina Castro's breakthrough and insightful personal story of her successful battle with stage IV lung cancer over twenty-four months offers information to cancer patients who face ordeals after being diagnosed with this storm. She describes this often-deadly disease from the perspective of a wise and proactive patient who specializes in art therapy as a means of finding her inner resources. Valentina emphasizes taking control and being skeptical about conventional medicine's triad of surgery, radiation therapy, and chemotherapy.

As an artist, she steps out of the box in the deep journey into her soul. In so doing, she rejects conventional protocols and, against objections from friends and relatives, searched for tailor-made treatments.

Lung cancer is the leading cause of cancer deaths in both men and women, accounting for over 150,000 deaths per year in the United States. The survival rate of stage IV adult cancers in the United States, as documented in the *Journal of Clinical Oncology*, at five years is a dismal 2.1 percent. A similar retrospective study in Australia has similar results of 2.3 percent survival.

Valentina describes her experience vividly in this book and mentions how she dealt with fear: "Even though you're terrified, you can get out of this."

The following examples are some of the many reactions I have witnessed in my patients for over forty-five years: Once the word *cancer* is mentioned, many patients feel blindsided and defeated. Any discussion beyond this is forgotten or not absorbed. Patients are often immobilized, unable to talk or walk. Multiple painful emotions come rushing forward: anger, denial, fear, self-pity, feeling cheated. In addition, there is often overwhelming worry of how other family members, friends, and business associates will handle the news.

Valentina clearly states, "Cancer won't define me."

Sometimes overwhelming panic and anxiety occur, causing insomnia, tremors, headaches, and scattered thoughts, along with nightmares regarding death.

Valentina experienced many of these emotions, but with a clear brain, she decided to seek my protocol, based on genomic testing of circulating tumor (stem) cells, followed by low-dose, insulin-potentiated chemotherapy over a three-week period.

Valentina describes her easy philosophy: "The mission of this life is to take good care of yourself."

Valentina describes in detail her personal journey in a poignant manner in order to help others undergoing the same trauma. One of the values of her book relates to her skepticism with conventional medicine and distrust of the system for which President Nixon declared, "War on cancer and over $200 billion has been spent in that effort—the results have been a supreme disappointment."

The side effects and adverse toxicities of surgery, radiation, and chemotherapy and after all three modalities are used can be devastating; even death can occur after the first course of full-dose chemotherapy. After two treatment cycles in November 2016 and March 2017, Valentina is enjoying a complete control with few side effects.

This book is a must-read for all newly diagnosed cancer patient and their families. She is to be congratulated for her courageous decisions.

—Dr. James Forsythe

Dr. Forsythe is a board-certified internist, medical oncologist, and homeopathic doctor and is board-eligible in pathology, gerontology, and anti-aging medicine. He has been an instructor of medicine at the University of California in San Francisco and an associate professor of medicine at the University of Nevada School of Medicine in Reno. He is an honorably retired full colonel in the US Army Medical Corps and served in South Vietnam, 1969–1970. He also was mobilized to serve in the Gulf War in Iraq prior to his retirement. He has authored or has chapters in over twenty-five books and is mentioned in Suzanne Somers's best-selling book Knockout: Interviews with Doctors Who Are Curing Cancer.

—⟨⟨⟩⟩—

Connie Solera:

When Valentina learned that she might have cancer, she asked if I had any reservations about her participating in my year-long artist-mentoring program called IGNITE. I told her that as long as her doctor approved, I would love to have her.

Her first biopsy was scheduled for what was also the first day of IGNITE. I assured Valentina it would be okay if she missed our meeting; she could always watch the recording later on. That morning, Valentina decided to listen to her inner guidance and postpone her procedure. Instead, she showed up to that first call of IGNITE, and our journey together began.

They say when the student is ready, the teacher will arrive. Valentina might have hired me to be her mentor that year, but she became one of my greatest teachers ever.

As an artist, I know first-hand how powerful the creative process is to fostering one's emotional, mental, and spiritual well-being. That year, Valentina showed me that the creative process can also save one's life—literally.

When I think back on our time together in IGNITE, I remember how Valentina still attended our meetings, even during her darkest moments. The fear I felt in my own heart was overwhelming when I saw Valentina's sunken face and IVs staring back at me.

But Valentina never complained. I never heard her once say "Why me?" or "I can't do this." She simply showed up again and again, using her own inner compass and ruthless determination to navigate her journey with cancer, hoping to one day help others do the same.

Valentina beat the odds that were stacked against her because she chose to believe in herself, her body's wisdom, and the healing power of creativity. I know this because I received the incredible honor of walking beside her on this path.

What you are holding in your hands today is not just a book; it is a sunken treasure that Valentina bravely dived to the depths of her own heart to discover and now shares with all of us who are seeking deep healing and that sense of aliveness that we, as humans, deserve.

May Valentina's wisdom and courage bless and inspire you as much as it has me.

May you be well.

—Connie Solera
January 2019

Connie Solera is an artist, teacher, and traveler with a mission to inspire every woman to pick up her paintbrush, let go her fears, and sink into the artist her heart is calling her to be. Through international retreats, online workshops, and her colorful, soulful art, Connie guides women on adventures of creative self-discovery to claim their power as artists. To learn more about Connie Solera visit www.ConnieSolera. com and @ConnieSolera on Instagram.

"If there is a book that you want to read
but it hasn't been written yet,
you must be the one to write it"

Toni Morrison

INTRODUCTION

I might have everything settled in my life, other than my struggle with cancer. Cancer is not an easy entertainment. It is intangible, though it's something that was in my mind, spirit, and body for a while. It's hard to learn to live and deal with it, at least for a period, because it is my intention to eradicate it from my system once and for all.

Nevertheless, I've been living with a huge question mark over my shoulders. There are a lot of unanswered questions: What is the sense of life? We must have a sense of life, but what's the sense of having sense? Making money? Why should we need to buy stuff? Who is in charge of setting life's lodestones besides my own lodestones? God? A system? Who pulls the strings?

I believe that each human being in this world has a reality, an ego that dictates his or her life. We each undoubtedly think that we know the truth of everything, and we are eager to fight for our truths. Is it really worth it? Or is it only the ego, hungry for victory? What about our spirit? These questions bring me to ask myself, *Then what is love? What is fear?* They are opposite energies, but the good thing is that we have the power to choose between them. And the most important thing to know is that love is on the other side of fear.

If you're wondering how this can be possible, that is exactly what this book is about. Thinkers, theorists, psychologists, poets, and artists throughout the world's history have tried to find answers to their personal questions, and most of them have found both issues and solutions. But to be honest, I think that nothing is real! Everything is a personal assumption and illusion.

Regardless, in my experience with cancer and as a healer and art therapist, the clue was to find out what was the reason of it in my life. What did I need to learn through the illness and/or the healing process? (What do you need to learn?)

This "thinking storm" at the end is for good. I might not have the correct answers, but I learned to accept myself, and that has been quite helpful. The more I accept myself, the less I need to feel accepted by others. Who cares about others' opinions anyway?

I have learned to be compassionate to myself, to have self-acceptance, and to be delighted in my eccentricity, in my greatness. We all are eccentric and have greatness in our ways. It requires courage to survive storms (illness, anxiety, panic attacks, divorce). We all have our particular storms to deal with, and standing firm in the face of adversity is necessary, as well as having determination, responsibility, and endurance for all kind of encounters.

But overall, the knowledge and understanding of the concept of unity and alignment have been a crucial ingredient in my healing process. Also, empathy, kindness, and unconditional love are emotions so needed to find the way to calm my inner storm. Each storm is valid and deserves to be honored.

It is my goal through this book to guide you through your storms and to go across the bridge of fear to find the love you deserve on the other side. Healing is a process, and it can be a loving (although a bit bumpy) journey to your recovery. It's an opportunity to make peace with yourself by changing your limiting beliefs and getting rid of some ghosts.

I promise there is a beautiful place inside you, where your essence (your truth) is waiting. Stop looking outside for solutions!

If I could, you can!

Part I

THE TURNING POINT

Chapter 1

HOW COULD THIS HAPPEN TO ME?

> *For the meaning of life differs from man to man, from day to day and from hour to hour. What matters, therefore, is not the meaning of life in general but rather the specific meaning of a person's life at a given moment.*
> —Viktor E. Frankl

Even though You're Terrified, You Can Get Out of This!

I knew that something was wrong with my health for around six months. I was fatigued, irritable; I slept for only a few hours and skipped some meals. I always felt stressed and tried to multitask family, housekeeping duties, and patients in my art therapy practice. I began coughing, but I thought it was due to allergies because it was that time of the year when pollen is all over the place. When I went out of town, and the cough didn't stop.

Before that, my recurring thoughts were related more to frustration, fear, and sometimes despair. Not everything was that bad; it's just that my attention and thoughts were leaning toward that energy: fear. It could be fear of failure, of illness, of losing a loved one, or of death. These kinds of thoughts are present in almost all human beings; it's part of being human. I'll talk about fear in greater detail later in this book because it is crucial to understand the meaning of it and its effect on our bodies, minds, and emotions.

1

However, despite being terrified, it is possible to move on. Moreover, it is possible to get ahead and learn to handle the situations of life that generate that fear, terror, or impotence. And turn that emotion around to find peace and balance in your mental and physical health. You can even get to the point of being acutely aware of the present moment and make your life a life that matters.

Once you achieve this skill, you will be able to redirect your path to walk through the purpose of your life and your truth. It might sound like magic or nearly impossible, but most people keep seeking throughout their lives for something that's missing. We might look desperately everywhere—workshops, retreats, books, religions, etc.—but, my dear reader, I must tell you this: that emptiness, that fear, those answers that you're looking for are within you, but you're too busy doing stuff, wanting someone to magically solve your life as soon as possible (and painlessly, if we can ask for more). And if that someone does not arrive, then you feel anxious and terrified.

Some people think that by making others see their mistakes, it will make them better, but they don't realize that they're trying to fix the outside while avoiding fixing what is happening on the inside. It's an ego trap. (More on the role of the ego in the healing process later in this book.) Thus, pointing out someone else's mistakes serves as justification for not assuming responsibility, and there is nothing easier than playing the role of the archetype of the victim, which is also terrifying. But who sees them as mistakes? What is perfection? Everything is relative, including time. None of them can be controlled; as a matter of fact, it's easier to learn how to manage your life than to control it. Let me tell you something—the lack of control can be terrifying as well.

You might think that this could be just another random book on your bookshelf, but it could be more than that. Nevertheless, this book offers a series of techniques and exercises that I have found useful in overcoming fear (I suffered from panic attacks after my diagnosis), as well as answers to many questions. I know this could work for you simply because I am alive to write this book for you. Against all the odds, after a diagnosis of lung cancer, I kept my both lungs. I learned to reconnect to the wisdom of the self-healing power of my body. I discovered these tips and have been using them successfully, as have others, so my desire is to share this information with you.

I became my own best advocate. I became my healer. I am positive you can overcome fear and become your best advocate and your own healer because no one knows your body better than you do.

Confirming the Diagnosis Can Be Stressful, Painful, and Overwhelming

Receiving a cancer diagnosis or a diagnosis of any disease that is potentially terminal is terrifying. When I received the lung cancer diagnosis, it freaked me out! It was literally a bio-shock; all my cells and my entire body was affected in that moment. My heartbeat was faster than ever, my breathing was burning my throat, and my body was shaking. It was similar to when I'd been assaulted at gunpoint; I could feel every pore of my skin.

A sequence of memories ran in my head in fast motion, and I even envisioned future events. I saw myself in my coffin, looking out at my husband, my children, my parents, my siblings, and my dearest friends, all surrounding me and weeping.

At that moment, fear officially controlled me. Nevertheless, I tried hard to calm down and pull myself together. In fact, outwardly, I was pretty cool. I was aware of the response of my mind, body, and spirit, but I explained to myself that everything was going to be okay. I told myself I needed to see a specialist because in a family clinic, the staff wasn't qualified to give that diagnosis to anyone. *How can they say such a thing after only one x-ray?* I thought. *I need more proof.* I denied my reality.

I felt the diagnosis was thrown in my face, as if the doctor was congratulating me on a hoped-for pregnancy. The doctor had a fake smile frozen on her pale face. I felt like a robot was giving me the diagnosis—so inhuman and lacking empathy, so absolutely heartless.

I understand that it's not easy to give this kind of bad news, but I do believe in empathy and compassion. Despite this negative experience, I knew from the bottom of my soul that everything was going to be okay. As a matter of fact, I promised that to myself. I pledged it to myself.

I called my husband as soon as I left the clinic and told him to meet me at home. He knew something was wrong, so he made me tell him the news over the phone. I hated to do that; it seemed I was the same robot, giving such news to my beloved husband. I couldn't find the words; they were all packed in my throat, but somehow, I spit them out.

When I arrived home, he was waiting for me in the living room. He hugged me; no words needed. I could tell he had cried before I got home.

After that day, life was a roller coaster for my family and me. Too many ups and downs and many adventures—lab work, CT scans, PET scans, x-rays, emotions, tears, and tough decisions. But believe it or not, there also was laughter, love, and gratitude. Overall, this journey has been a huge transformation. We've been back and forth to doctor appointments in Houston, where I live (although I have to confess that visiting MD Anderson Cancer Center in Houston was not my cup of tea), and in Reno, Nevada, where my doctor is.

I'm not the same Valentina as I was before cancer. It seems that I was meant to experience a transformation. Although I encountered difficult moments, I never thought I would resign. No way! I am not that easy!

Still, it has been quite a journey. Fear is a horrible emotion/energy; it can consume anyone. Despite that, there always was hope and faith in the depths of my heart. I think that the key is to bring light to darkness. I found that light (faith) through meditation. Meditation is my sacred moment. I found a way to connect to the divine within me—we all have this ability. (More on that concept in the following chapters.) Cancer transformed my life for the better in many ways. Cancer was my awakening call.

Cancer Won't Define Me

After I received my diagnosis, I visited several doctors. I first went to a pulmonologist, who was as surprised as my husband and I were, as I have always been a very healthy person. He couldn't understand why I was there, as my file seemed "clean," but he had not seen my x-ray and CT scan results. When he read through them, his face changed. How could a young woman (forty-six years old) have lung cancer when she is not a smoker and has no family history of cancer?

He ordered a variety of tests to check that diagnosis. First, he pulled almost one liter of fluid from my left lung. The liquid was clear, which was a good sign, because when there is cancer, a color is evident. At that moment, we had some peace of mind, but as I was leaving the imaging office, I suddenly couldn't breathe, and I felt a sharp pain in my lung area. The nurses immediately brought a wheelchair and took me back to the exploration room.

That was my first experience in dealing with pain while simultaneously dealing with an out-of-control situation. Somehow, I was able to stabilize my condition on my own, which was fortunate because the doctors could not do anything—my vital signs didn't show any abnormalities. What had happened was that my lung had reshaped to its size and natural form.

I experienced the power of the mind taking care of pain and bringing calm as I returned to my center. It was a practice I had learned in hypnobirthing training, which I took for two of my four pregnancies. I was amazed at how intuitively I handled this scary situation. This, however, was just the tip of the iceberg.

A couple of weeks later, I had a bronchoscopy and then a PET scan. A month after the initial diagnosis, it was confirmed. It was the longest and scariest month of my life. As soon as I read the results, I was devastated, scared, angry at God, and angry at myself. I kept asking, *Why me? How could this happen to me?* I was pretty sure I was a good person. I took care of my family and my clients. I volunteered with a group of immigrant women. I was always ready to help or do something for others. Why was God—or life—punishing me?

The truth is, though, that I didn't take care of the most important person in my life: *me*. (But I realized that after several months later and you will read about in in chapter 2). I began to have panic attacks— I have to confess that it was one of the worst things I've experienced in my entire life.

Now I had a huge mountain to climb, my personal Everest. I was referred to an oncologist, who was nice, but he could not hide his astonishment at the diagnosis in a woman of my age and with the health characteristics I had. He explained the steps we would follow: three rounds of chemotherapy, with a general medicine used to treat several types of cancer that had similar characteristics. After that, there would be a set of radiation.

I was shocked. Something inside me was shouting, *This is not what I need! This is not the way to heal!*

On my second visit, my mother and a friend came with me, and the oncologist told my mom that I was a "such a sad case." I couldn't believe he'd said that! He continued explaining the treatment I was supposed to follow, but I interrupted him to say, "Never, *ever* again say that I am 'a sad case.'" On the contrary, I wanted him to see me as a success story because I needed a doctor who could support me and give me the strength and faith to move on.

He wanted me to visit a thoracic surgeon, who was, he said, "the most expensive acquisition" of a known hospital in my area. The surgeon was the director of the Lung Cancer Institute in that hospital.

When I got there, the surgeon tested the function of my respiratory system and discovered it was at 50 percent of its capacity. Then he went through my paperwork and showed us, with his very fancy, expensive, state-of-art equipment, why he needed to remove my entire lung. Again, I heard my body shouting, *This is not what I need! This is not the way to heal!*

In that very moment, instead of freaking out, I felt something igniting inside me. It was a strange force. Suddenly, I felt brave.

I understood later that what I was feeling was courage and a determination to make my own decisions about my health and my body. I wasn't going to surrender to the medical system just because they had the medical knowledge. Don't get me wrong; I honor and respect doctors, but in a fraction of a second, I visualized myself in surgery, and I saw the surgeon tossing my lung into the trashcan. I felt goosebumps! No way!

Of course, my husband and I looked for second and third opinions. We went to another well-known cancer center in my area, where I visited another and very well-known thoracic surgeon. He said that my case was a "bad luck case." (*What's with the doctors?* I thought.) He also said that Mexicans, which is my ethnicity, tend to "turn to voodoo," referring to alternative medicine. He was Swiss, so culturally, maybe he thought there was a big difference in the way to approach health.

I also visited another oncologist, but she didn't want to go through my file. She asked me to have a biopsy before she could share an opinion.

Then I saw a specialist in infectious diseases. I wanted to know his point of view, but I hit a wall again.

Houston is known as the mecca of cancer treatment; people come from all over the world to be treated there. In my case, however, going to the cancer center was my worst nightmare. That place made me feel like I was in Disneyland for cancer—a place where you can find all kinds of souvenirs related to cancer. It was certainly not the happiest place on earth for me: an overwhelming reassurance of the dark side of my health situation. The marketing was overwhelming aswell. The vibe and energy that I felt there was so heavy that I could barely breathe. The atmosphere was so depressing for me that it made me feel that the place was fake. It was like entering an endless spiral controlled by the medical system and the pharmaceutical industry, and they were in charge of moving the strings of the patients; it was a monster that needs patients to survive until it sucks them to death.

What's more, I felt like a character from Aldous Huxley's *Brave New World*, where you are programmed to be happy and to heal but according to the convenience of the system. I felt lonely and hopeless, fighting against a giant. (The cancer center works amazingly for many people, but this is my personal opinion.)

I refused to be part of it! I refused to become a number. I refuse to be part of their statistics. I refused to be defined by cancer. I refused to give away my power. I knew, deep down in my heart, that we all have wisdom and a capacity for self-healing. It's teamwork: patient and doctor.

Have You Been Overdiagnosed?

Once you are diagnosed, a new door opens, and with it, the roller coaster accelerates. You can feel it in the pit of your stomach. Your mind can't understand what is going on around you, and you receive so much information that it's hard to register everything. It's like stepping into a bottomless barrel; everything the doctors and their staff tell you is overwhelming. At least, that's how it seemed to me. As soon as I started treatment, information about my diagnosis continued to emerge. Instead of feeling that I was beginning to solve the problem with the treatment, it was the other way around. Rather than seeing the light at the end of the tunnel, it was becoming darker and endless.

I was so afraid, clueless, and powerless that I decided to trust my oncologist 100 percent. I simply delivered all the responsibility to him. I had no ounce of energy to make any decision.

I began my first round of chemo, and it went okay. Then there was the second one, and after that, I started feeling too weak, too out of my center. I had one left, though. Between the second and third treatment, I decided to finish the three-round treatment, but something in the bottom of my heart began to awake. I decided I was done with this chemo thing.

Before cancer, I always understood the correlation between mind, body, and spirit. I was very intrigued and read lots of books about it. After the second chemo, I was clear about the dissociation between mind, body, and spirit. I could feel discomfort in my body, but my mind couldn't register exactly where. My spirit wanted to run away from my body because it was as if it did not recognize it anymore as its vehicle to be transported in this life. My mind once again was struggling to convince that fugitive spirit to stay in whatever it chose as its abode. This situation ignited my inner voice; it ignited the beginning of the communication and consciousness between my voice and me. I became aware.

Meanwhile, I visited a cancer center for other opinions and continued visiting my oncologist, who was aware of my movements. I realized then that the system (the Big Brother) was following my steps. Everything was in my file—every doctor I visited, every IV I had, every test, every pill, everything. I had no place to hide. I felt trapped and without outlet, destined to follow the indications of others. Who or what was I, then? And what about my needs? My emotions? My decisions? My intuition? My freedom?

I understand that every patient responds differently to treatments, but I felt like a lab rat. No doctor ever asked me anything; they simply ordered studies and more studies. On one occasion, I refused to get an MRI because the doctor said that "by-the-book cancer" could have metastasized in my brain. I knew that, in my case, it would not happen like that (my voice told me that), and I refused to do the MRI.

His response was, "I recommended you follow my instructions. I like you and don't want you to die because you are still young." (Again, seriously?)

From that moment, I felt that I needed to be on the defensive at every appointment in case he threw a bomb, based on his going by the book.

To make matters worse, despite the fear of death that cancer carries, scientific literature—for instance, in the *Journal of the National Cancer Institute*—shows the statistics of "overdiagnosis" in patients with breast and lung cancer. By overdiagnosis, it is known as a cancer diagnosis but without symptoms or death; so in the search of a diagnosis, all kind of nonesential studies could be done or prescirbed. In this case, cancer may not be treated clinically; it could regress spontaneously. Sometimes patients may be treated with unnecessary procedures that deplete the quality of life.

For instance, when my doctor wanted to remove my lung, he argued that it was necessary to prevent a metastasis, and that I also needed a series of radiation treatments to control the cancer. I wonder what my quality of life would have been if I had blindly followed his suggestions. Thank God, my inner voice was much louder. From there, I decided to listen to my inner voice because I discovered that it is wise. There was no one better than my inner voice to guide me, so I decided to fire my oncologist, and I resigned from the conventional medical system. It was one of the most difficult but most fortunate decisions in my cancer-healing process.

What Is Fear?

Our bodies have different systems, one of which is the anatomic nervous system (ANS), considered a self-control system which intrinsically is tied to the peripheral nervous system (PNS). It basically regulates the internal environment of the body, exchanging commands between the PNS and organs in order to maintain vital body functions. There are two divisions in the ANS: the sympathetic nervous system and the parasympathetic nervous system. Both systems usually act on the same organ and generate the same action potentials, yet their functions are different and oppose each other.

The sympathetic nervous system prepares the body for emergency situations. The kind of fear related to these emergency situations is known as fight-or-flight response or stress response, which is a survival mechanism designed to put the body on full alert—in case you need to run away from attackers, for example. When you have a life-threatening event, fear is present to protect you. Fear is your hero, and it is a genuine fear.

In the other hand, the parasympathetic nervous system restores the organism to its normal position. This system is responsible for maintaining the activities such as rest and digest or feed and breed that occur when the body is at rest. However, nowadays the world is full of bad and stressing news, and this puts us in survival mode, twenty-four/seven. Having access to information (good and bad) at our fingertips limits our bodies' ability to find the right balance for optimal performance. Our warning mechanisms begin to fail, making us feel unsure and, therefore, fearful.

In reality, fear is conceived in our imaginations. It is a fictitious fear, but we live it as very real because our brains are not able to distinguish between a genuine and a fictitious fear, to the extent that it can lead to a physical or mental illness.

But what if fear shows up in your life as a messenger? Then you may want to stop and listen to the message, instead of running from it. These words can be limiting beliefs about money, health, work, or relationships. Fear acts as an alert of something that needs to be addressed, and that's the message.

How are we to distinguish between genuine and fictitious fear? That is the challenge. Genuine fear is related to real things, such as emergencies, heartbreaking events, and so forth, and fictitious fear is related to our imaginations, when we make up a story about a real situation.

Remember how the sympathetic nervous system acts and that it results in a genuine fear. Fictitious fear, in turn, works with the parasympathetic nervous system.

Why is this information necessary for you? Well, when you received a cancer diagnosis, in the first moment, you experience a genuine fear. Your body responds to an immediate life-threating event. It could last several minutes. But after that, you begin to experience a fictitious fear because after the trauma of receiving the news of the disease, your mind starts to imagine a series of things related to stress and even death. It is very likely that you will have panic attacks throughout the day (or night) for an extended period. These attacks are a consequence of your imagination, and therefore, you will live like a slave of your own fictitious fear. That is why it is crucial to distinguish between one fear and the other so you can manage panic attacks and even make them disappear.

Chapter 2

MOVING FROM "WHY ME?" TO "WHAT FOR?"

Courage is resistance to fear, mastery of fear, not absence of fear.
—Mark Twain

What Are Those Voices inside Your Head?

We all have a constant voice in our minds—sometimes more than one—that is an internal dialogue with ourselves. This voice either guides us or scolds us. It is a natural conversation, but what or who is this voice? Some people call it intuition; others refer to it as the self. This definition depends on whether you are an analytical person or one more prone to spirituality. Inevitably, neurologists differ because they tend to seek the physical location where this phenomenon generates. However, this voice has an explanation from the neuroscientific point of view; it is based on thoughts. The voice has a fundamental influence on the physiological balance of the brain and, therefore, on our health, including our destinies.

Beyond our genetics, a theory has been discovered in the last decades on the effect our thinking has on our lives. The simple idea that you can change your life by changing your beliefs is fascinating. Our society has existed for thousands of years, and we have been taught to be victims of destiny instead of being co-creators of it. Isn't this amazing?

Science now recognizes that the fate and behavior of an organism is directly linked to its perception of the environment.

In simple terms, the nature of our lives is based on how we perceive it. To go deeper into the subject, *epigenetics* is the science of how environmental signals select, modify, and regulate gene activity. This new awareness reveals that our genes are constantly remodeled in response to life experiences, which again emphasizes that our perception of life shapes our biology.

It is imperative to be aware of the type of dialogue we hold with ourselves, as well to be conscious of our environment because the thoughts generated by our belief system are the watershed to build or destroy our lives. The insights we gain through this new biology unleash the power of consciousness, matter, and miracles. (In chapter 5, I'll discuss how changing your beliefs can change your life to the point that you can be your own healer.)

Handling Panic Attacks and Fear of Dying

Some research suggests that our bodies' natural fight-or-flight response to danger could be involved in panic or anxiety attacks. For instance, if a lion comes after you, your body would react instinctively. Your heart rate and breathing would speed up as your body prepared itself for a life-threatening situation. Many of the same reactions occur in a panic attack, but it's not known why a panic attack happens when no obvious danger is present. The danger is present because we perceive it as such, even though there is no apparent reason for it.

Panic attacks typically begin abruptly without warning. They can strike at any time—when you're driving a car, at the mall, sound asleep, or in the middle of a business meeting. You may have occasional panic attacks, or they may occur frequently. Panic-attack symptoms may include a sense of impending doom or danger; fear of loss of control or death; a rapid, pounding heart rate; sweating; shaking; shortness of breath or tightness in your throat; or chills, among others. One of the worst things about a panic attack is the intense fear that you'll have another one because they are unpredictable. You may fear having a panic attack so much that you avoid situations where they may occur.

In my case, panic attacks paralyzed me. Usually, the attacks came while I was watching TV or sleeping. They began with a sound that came from outside my house, as if the earth crunched—like the sound of the creaking of the earth during an earthquake. That was the sign that a panic attack was approaching. Then I would see a shadow on the floor that began to surround me, a dense darkness that approached me, little by little. At that moment, I felt cold to the extent of freezing and felt paralyzed. It became harder to breathe, and my heart beat with a force that I had never felt.

This was a tough situation to handle; my mind was totally out of control. I felt like the shadow was swallowing me. It was as if I were sinking into quicksand and was completely unarmed. Fortunately, my husband always realized when I had panic attacks, and he helped me get out of that state with exactly the right words and unconditional love. I will always be grateful for that.

For many years in my professional practice, I was able to help my patients who suffered from panic attacks. I led them, step by step, out of the whirlwind. But it was not until I received the diagnosis of cancer, which confronted me with death, that I began to have panic attacks. My mind created everything, but at the same time, my mind could no longer handle it. It was an endless spiral.

How was I able to break that vicious circle generated by my mind? How did I defeat that shadow that appeared to devour me and steal my peace? Well, I will reveal it throughout this book.

Meditation (Stillness of Mind)

Through meditation, I feel that I belong to everything, and everything belongs to me. There is no space for judgment. I can see and feel through other eyes—the eyes of compassion. I don't need to sit in a particular position when I am meditating (though I must sit straight); I just focus on my breathing. Although I do that to exercise my lungs, meditation can be practiced while walking, running, being in nature, listening to your favorite music and/or mantras, dancing, laughing, or making love—anything that is a stress-reliever activity. It's as simple as being present in the moment.

If you like creative activities, like painting, coloring, writing, art journaling, etc., art is a fantastic way to address all kind of emotions. I see no other effective way to realize so many things happening in my life at the same time; many of them cannot be expressed in words. Once in a while, I need so desperately to let go of all the reflection and the process that is going on in my soul, mind, and body. I need to pour it somewhere so that I can observe it from a different perspective—from the outside. I don't know what would become of me without art. Creativity is a natural state of all human beings. Creativity is a tool for the healing process. (More information on that in chapter 7.)

There are many things in life that are beyond our control, but we can take responsibility for our states of mind and change them for the better. This is the most important thing we can do; it is the only real antidote to our personal sorrows and to the anxieties, fears, hatred, and general confusion that beset the human condition.

Meditation is a means of transforming the mind. Different meditation techniques encourage and develop concentration, clarity, emotional positivity, and a calm seeing of the true nature of things. By engaging in a particular meditation practice, you learn the patterns and habits of your mind. The practice offers a means to cultivate new, more positive ways of being. With regular work and patience, these healthy, focused states of mind can deepen into profoundly peaceful and energized states of mind. Such experiences can have a transformative effect and can lead to a new understanding of life.

It can be very challenging to find the peace and time to create the habit of meditation. The first step is the hardest.

Meditation saved my life. It helped me to stop the vicious circle. I found my inner peace but overall, through meditation I changed my limiting beliefs. I was feeling trapped by my negative thoughts and fears, but I was able to cross that barrier that gave me the opportunity to return to live life with hope and to find my life purpose.

Today, I still meditate because it is the best way to start the day. And it has become a habit. I focus on the positive and set my daily intention, as well as aligning my mind and my heart.

How to Trust Your Intuition

What is intuition? By definition, it has six different aspects:

1. direct perception of truth, fact, etc., independent of any reasoning process; immediate apprehension
2. a fact, truth, etc., perceived in this way
3. a keen and quick insight
4. the quality or ability of having such direct perception or quick insight
5. philosophy
    a) an immediate cognition of an object not inferred or determined by a previous cognition of the same object
    b) any object or truth so discerned
    c) pure, untaught, non-inferential knowledge
6. *linguistics.* The ability of the native speaker to make linguistic judgments, as of the grammaticality, ambiguity, equivalence, or nonequivalence of sentences, deriving from the speaker's native-language competence.

Have you ever had a moment when you felt as though something wasn't right? Like your gut or something inside your body was talking to you? Perhaps you've stepped into an isolated or dark place and felt uneasy or felt negative about someone without knowing why? If you've experienced this, did you ignore it and dismiss it as illogical nonsense?

In some Eastern countries, this perception is normal, but in the West, it is not. As part of the Western culture, we have learned that rationality should predominate when making decisions about anything from practical business organizations to what to wear on a date. But what of that inner voice, that butterfly feeling, that struggle between our logical and analytical minds and our instinctive or intuitive knowledge buried in the body?

We live in constant conflict between reason and intuition throughout our lives in making the best decisions for work and family. This is what makes us different from animals; they are only instinctive. Finding the balance is hard, though we tend to be more rational most of the time because it makes us feel safer than using intuition as a guidance tool. Even though sometimes intuition speaks out loud, we become deaf!

If we pay attention to our inner voice, we are ashamed to admit that we followed that inner voice to make certain decisions. We can even be afraid of the power of intuition, which is the voice of our truths.

We don't credit that capacity, and we find a way to quiet our voices because sometimes it could be confrontational to listen to whatever it has to say. We become skeptical, and we rather mistrust ourselves; hence, we sabotage ourselves.

How can we seek balance? Find a way for intuition and the mind to make the peace. It sounds weird, but it is possible, and it can be easier than you might think.

Seven Tips to Ignite Your Intuition

1. Be aware of your feelings and thoughts; don't fight them. Go with the flow.
2. Center your attention in your body. Is it relaxed or stressed?
3. Listen to your favorite music; while listening visualize/imagine the music.
4. Go for a walk or run; be in contact with nature.
5. Write in your journal as a daily habit or do art journaling.
6. Listen to other people's stories. Be compassionate.
7. Read an inspiring book. Take notes, underline, draw—whatever comes to mind.

What about Skepticism?

Skepticism can become a discipline, a way of life. We can be skeptical about religion, government, ideologies, people, and so on. Lots of people defend their points of view without evidence but based on their stories, beliefs, and fears; that is to say, their own truths. Yet for everyday life (work, love, money, and health), the decisions are based on good evidence.

People can be skeptical (uncertain) about intuition because it is empirical, but they can be certain about the reason, as it is verifiable. Sometimes is convenient to be skeptical about our inner voice, which I see this like a tramp from ego. In other words, ego is trying to do everything possible to distract you from changing your mind.

Ego is always trying to win all the battles; it will do whatever is necessary to quiet our truths and automatically live our lives without taking any responsibility, in some cases. That's why we develop a habit of questioning whether the things we believe are real. These querying makes us let go of beliefs we have when things are not as we thought they were. Of course, we won't let go so quickly, and this is challenging. It requires discipline to give way to credibility but to understand that our bodies are able to heal themselves.

It does not mean that we will believe absolutely everything we are told. The most important thing is to stop being skeptical of the force that has our intuition, which is never wrong. Then we will have to silence the mind and trust in ourselves, and for this, we need to be aware and awakened.

Mile 8—the Beginning of an Infinite Journey

Although I do not consider myself a passionate runner, I started to run, motivated by my husband's passion—he's a runner and does it very well. I have run some 5K races, ten-mile races, and even a half marathon once, and I enjoyed it very much. I started training for a ten-mile race, and on the first day of training, I felt tremendously bad. I lacked air. I felt heavy and frustrated. But there was something inside me that told me to stop running and start walking; I was afraid because the message of my body had a connotation of danger. I got to the meeting point, where my fellow runners were waiting for me. I arrived much later than everyone.

That day coincided with the week in which I expected the results of my x-rays and the fatal diagnosis. As soon as I learned my diagnosis, I advised my colleagues that, for health reasons, I was withdrawing from the training, but I continued to participate as a cheerleader for them in a group online chat.

One day before the race, one of the members of the team sent an email to all of us. In it, she shared to whom she was dedicating each mile. To my surprise, mile number 8 was dedicated to me. I'd met this person on the first day of the training, but we continued in to have contact through group chat. I was very touched. From that moment, all my companions joined the plan, and since then, in all the races in which they still run as a team, they dedicate mile 8 to me.

Curiously enough, after few days, I made the association between the number eight and the symbol for infinity. It coincided with my birthday, and I received several gifts, including two necklaces and a pair of earrings with the symbol of infinity. I took this coincidence as a kind of sign.

My inner voice told me to go deeper into the concept of infinity. What I saw was a relationship between mind, body, and spirit. This may be controversial because some cultures do not believe that life ends with death, but as far as I am concerned, this was the guideline to delve into what is undoubtedly my mission in life.

I have the understanding that the body is a vehicle to travel in this life and that the soul has pending subjects to learn, but what are these subjects? I do not know! For that, I am here to learn. For that, we are all here, only some people have not discovered that they are learning from the experiences and life stories in which they somehow have chosen to be. And they have not taken responsibility for learning.

Other people, have understood this responsibility for the good. And others, like me, for "the bad". It took cancer to have me understand that I must learn: yes or yes! Although one day a doctor told me that my case was "bad luck," I see it as good luck because I have been forced into the classroom of life to learn to live in my mission and my purpose in life. Cancer was my wake-up call.

Before my diagnosis, I used to live, and after it, I existed. As Descartes said, "I think, therefore I am." This reflection began at mile 8, and I know it will transcend through time into different bodies and different life histories.

The Mission in This Life Is to Take Good Care of Yourself

As I've said, I understood my mission of life, and I dare say that mission is the mission of every human being—taking care of ourselves. What can be more important than ourselves? It's not about being selfish and stepping over everyone, but it is about being *healthily selfish*. That is, we must know how to put up healthy boundaries, when necessary; take care of our nutrition and rest; express ourselves with freedom; and respect ourselves and others. Look in the mirror, and accept and love the person who is reflected in it. Walk with a steady step and with the certainty that, whatever the destination, your mission will arrive as a whole. Our bodies are our temples and deserve to be treated like a sacred place. We need to understand healthy self-esteem, healthy nutrition, healthy spirit, and healthy thoughts.

Loving our neighbor also is part of taking care of ourselves, as well as being grateful to others. Speaking from the heart to others is speaking to yourself from the heart. Helping others with compassion is being compassionate with ourselves. Altruism implicitly carries a second profit, and in many cases, much more is received than we can give.

That is why, my dear friend, the more that you care, protect, and love yourself, the more your mission in life will make sense. You will establish a deep contact with your being, and this will be extended outward. The most important relationship in your life is with yourself because, in turn, this connects you with your spirit and with the divine, beyond any religious belief or dogma. Therefore, you will achieve inner peace.

Maybe this sounds like illogical or irrational; I was talking about skepticism earlier. Remember that your ego may be in alert mode. Maybe it does make sense, but you do not know where or how to achieve inner peace.

My desire is that you will be able to unite in this concept of love and respect for yourself. Therefore, the closest relationship with your spirituality, which is understanding the Divine whinin; and enjoying existence pass through in this life. Without drama and in harmony with yourself. You will find your mile 8—the beginning of your journey.

Part II

HEALING YOUR FOUR BODIES: PHYSICAL, EMOTIONAL, MENTAL, AND SPIRITUAL

Chapter 3

UNDERSTANDING YOUR PHYSICAL BODY

Do not fear the lack of knowledge, fear false knowledge.
—Leo Tolstoy

Researching Cancer

Do you sometimes have a discomfort in your body, but you don't always know what it is? Are you a workaholic? Do you skip meals? Do you exercise too much or not at all? Do you drink or smoke too much? Do you use drugs? In a nutshell, do you abuse your body?

Sometimes we take our bodies for granted and assume they will endure whatever we do to it, but that is not so. Our bodies have a limit. The body is an incredible machine, but it deserves respect. It is our temple. In the last chapter I spoke of the body as our vehicle and that it deserves maintenance. You have to be aware of gasoline level so you can move and oil to work in optimum conditions; in short, it's worthy of the care we would give to a luxury car. It's important for you to know what is necessary about your vehicle.

There is latent cancer within each of us. Our bodies continuously generate flawed cells, and this is how tumors occur. However, our bodies are provided with a series of mechanisms to detect and block these types of cells. The body's defense mechanisms prevent more catastrophic results than the statistics suggest—one person out of four.

When you have a diagnosis of cancer, it is crucial to learn everything you can to help your body defend itself in the face of this disease. The body has the capacity and wisdom to heal itself, but in our Western culture, we do not have that awareness. We assume that if we stuff ourselves with medication, that will heal our bodies. We do need medicine to help the body—that's unquestionable—but if we abuse it, we will suppress the self-healing power of our bodies, particularly if we are aware that we are billions of cells packed into a body.

Most conventional doctors do not see the body as a whole but rather as independent sections. They do not have a holistic view of the body. For this reason, there are specialties: obstetricians, oncologists, ophthalmologists, etc., which gives them a limited vision of the body. From my point of view, it is essential to understand that every cell in the body is related to the others; for example, what happens in the digestive system is directly related to what happens to the skin. Have you ever eaten something that caused a skin reaction?

If you are reading this book, I assume it's because you have been diagnosed with cancer, or you're dealing with a chronic illness. Regardless of where the disease is located or the stage of it, you must assume the responsibility of making a drastic and immediate change in your habits.

It is possible that your oncologist (if you have one) will not notify you that you should avoid sugar, or tell you of the benefits of exercise, or say how crucial is the state of mind in which you find yourself to face the challenge of a diagnosis of this magnitude.

When I was diagnosed, I questioned my doctor on how I should change my habits, to which he replied, "If you want to, you could eat less red meat." That was it. He did not tell me anything else. Once again, however, my inner voice—my intuition—guided me to find the answers for myself on what I had to do to help my body to improve—to stop the inflammatory process, to level my pH, to detoxify, etc., everything that favored my health or inhibited the tendency of the characteristics of cancer.

And why don't most oncologists give you this information?

a) They have no idea because it is not scientifically tested, according to the norms that govern conventional medicine.

b) Oncology is a very complex field; it can hardly be up-to-date with advances in diagnostic and treatment research.

c) The pharmaceutical industry does not agree to have patients discover elsewhere how to find a cure for their illness.

d) Doctors have a warped view of the holistic functioning of the body.

e) Insurers would go bankrupt if the clients took control of their health and used the alternative route.

f) All of the above.

Understanding Your Body

Although there is much research and many advances in the science of medicine, especially in the field of cancer, most of it has been done with rats; it can take a long time for developments to be tested in humans. To get the appropriate medicine based on the results of such research can take years—and that's without considering what is required to design the protocols of treatments. With cancer, time has a disadvantage, as there are cases in which the patient is against the clock.

Faced with this situation, our hands are tied. However, we must focus on the fact that our bodies are the core resource for healing. As I've mentioned, the body has an innate wisdom. For example, when a baby has a fever, it's because the defense mechanism that is fighting a bacterium or virus has been activated. And what do adults do? We administer medication to help lower the fever, which suppresses the function of the baby's immune system. That is, we send the army to sleep, to nullify it. Of course, sometimes we administer the medication because we are afraid that a high temperature will bring worse consequences. But in general terms, that is our tendency—to prevent the body from doing what it does naturally.

And so from an early age, the body is inhibited and accustomed to not fulfilling its function. After a time of this constant interruption of its functions, the cells are conditioned to receive medication and become lazy. This is a consequence of a culture of a mass belief.

We all have latent cancer in our bodies, but our defense mechanisms act when a tumor occurs. And how do we activate these mechanisms? We begin by becoming aware of this simple fact: we are designed for self-healing. It's imperative that we learn how it works so that we can support it to fulfill its mission.

Nutrition: You Are What You Eat

In earlier times, people grew their own food, and it was customary to prepare food from scratch in the kitchen. People who lived on farms with animals knew that the animals would become food for the family. Kitchen utensils were made of natural materials, such as clay and wood. Over time, societies became more active and stopped spending so much time on food preparation to make way for frozen food and chemical preservatives, and fast food, microwave ovens, Teflon for avoiding cleaning time, etc. The containers in which food is sold and stored are made of plastic, derived from petroleum, a toxic agent that influences our food and therefore our bodies. That is why it is now recommended to use BPA-free plastics (BPA stands for bisphenol A, an industrial chemical that has been used to make certain plastics and resins since the 1960s and is found in polycarbonate plastics and epoxy resins[1]) to lessen the damage.

Another major problem has been global overpopulation, which forced the need to produce fruits, vegetables, and cereals throughout the year, when previously, there were only certain fruits per season. In trying to accelerate the continuous and massive production of these products, the industry has been forced to modify the soil (the famous GMO) and to use fertilizers, pesticides, etc. Cattle, chickens, and pigs are fed hormones and are exposed to antibiotics. Fish are

---

[1] http://www.mayoclinic.org/healthy-lifestyle/nutrition-and-healthy -eating/expert-answers/bpa/faq-20058331.

raised on farms, where they are also exposed to a kind of artificial production.

Do you realize what you are eating? Have you done any reflection about this? Do you know if what you give your body is artificial or natural? It's not my intention to provoke paranoia or any anxiety or panic attack, but it is *very* important that you are aware of what you eat.

When I started researching the kind of food I needed to give my body to help it, I was not completely aware of what it meant to nurture. I have never been one to overeat, but I didn't give much thought to the origin of what I ate. But pushed by my intuition after my diagnosis, I knew that food could be my best medicine. As I was researching, I became more aware of my nutrition, and I felt much better. (Later in this book, I will give you a list of books that propose diet as a way of healing.)

Nutrition does not only apply to what we eat; there is another type of nutrition that has to do with how we nourish our hearts. How do we manage our time or spend a good moment with ourselves? It is important to know what fills our souls—a hobby, a good book, quality time with family and friends, exercise, healthy relationships at work and home. Are you in balance with the things that nourish you?

It is also important to be aware of our states of mind when we sit down to eat. If we argue while we eat, or if we are in a depressive state, for example, this directly affects our bodies; many times, this incites eating disorders like anorexia and bulimia. The time that we dedicate to eating must be optimum so that our organisms realize the activity of digestion as such. As I mentioned earlier, we currently live against the clock. We go to fast-food restaurants, which are designed in such a way that people are not motivated to stay long so that the circulation of customers is frequent.

When I used to go to the oncologist, there was a big bowl of candies on the front desk—sugar! In the IV room, there was a bowl full of chocolates and one or two trays of cupcakes with colored icing. In other words, more sugar! I was alarmed and questioned the nurses, because cancer cells feed on sugar. It seemed Machiavellian to me! I even thought they did it on purpose so that clients would not heal, and they'd have captive clientele. But I prefer to think that the nurses never were taught about nutrition at nursing school, and that's why they allowed those sugar trays in the IV room.

Every time I questioned the nurses, they said the patients brought them to share, and that was "such a nice gesture."

I replied, "You must know the damage done to the body by excessive sugar and more so in patients with cancer. It is up to you to educate your patients."

Their only response was a frozen smile and a shrug.

On one occasion, I saw a patient drinking a Coke while she was talking on her cell phone and smoking a cigarette. I didn't judge her; my attention was focused on the level of unconscious, ignorance, or the comfort of not taking responsibility for oneself. (Okay, I might be a bit judgemental.)

Stop the Sugar and Cravings

Since sugar is the number-one enemy of cancer, I decided to remove it from my diet immediately: *zero refined sugar.* I stopped eating cakes, my sacred morning latte with its two tablespoons of sugar, chocolates, candies, bread, certain fruits like bananas, and so on. My decision was drastic! It was like deciding overnight to quit alcohol, smoking, or drugs.

Sugar generates addiction in the brain. In fact, many studies hold that sugar is now the worst drug of our time. And the worst of it is that the children are given sugar in tons every day: cookies, cakes, candies, sweeteners. The bombardment of marketing is constant.

Sugar addiction is real. Researchers at the Center for Obesity Prevention at Boston Children's Hospital designed the most sophisticated study to date, showing the stimulant effects of high-glycemic carbohydrates on the brain's centers of desire, reward, and hunger.

High-glycemic carbohydrates, such as sugar and white flour, are carbohydrates that produce rapid spikes and drops in blood sugar.

The results of the study, published in the *American Journal of Clinical Nutrition*, show how these foods, regardless of taste, intensely stimulate the same parts of the brain involved in drug addiction, altering the brain activity in a way that makes us experience even more cravings for these same foods. These results add more support to the controversial idea that food addiction, especially carbohydrates and sugar, is the real cause behind those who overeat.[2]

It is believed that the biological effects of refined carbohydrates, irrespective of their calories and taste, can lead to addiction-related symptoms, especially in susceptible people—those who are overweight or obese. If you think you might have a sugar addiction or you feel frustrated because of your uncontrollable cravings for sugary foods or because you can not lose weight, you might consider switching to a low-glycemic index diet (avoiding sugar, fruit juices, sweetened beverages, white rice, refined white flour, soft drinks, and other processed carbohydrates). This type of diet treats this addiction by stabilizing blood-sugar levels as it prevents abnormal fluctuations, and it does not activate the reward and desire systems of the brain. The result will be fewer cravings and less excessive hunger. Besides, high-glycemic index foods can be replaced with foods that contain more vitamins, minerals, fiber, and phytochemicals (substances found in foods of plant origin), which can fight many diseases, including cancer. I highly recommend seeing a nutritionist for further guidance.

Why Is It Important to Have an Anti-Cancer Diet?

Cancer is a disease with infinite dimensions for which only one intervention is rarely enough. It is necessary to combine several methods to be effective. There are natural methods that produce a

---

[2] https://universityhealthnews.com/daily/nutrition/sugar-addiction-new-study-validates-all-carb-calories-are-not-created-equal/

potent effect regarding angiogenesis (the growth of new capillary blood vessels in the body, is an important natural process used for healing and reproduction) and lack side effects and that can also combine with conventional therapies.

Good nutrition is imperative because many natural anti-angiogenesis (food that fight cancer) foods have been discovered. It's important to be aware of an anti-inflammatory method, (a diet that addresses inflammation) since the inflammation directly affects the growth of new tumors.

The immune system plays a significant role. It is composed of immune cells (NK killer cells –which are central components of the innate immunity, among others). These cells represents the chemical equipment that cuts cancer from its source. So everything that strengthens the immune system weakens the growth of cancer. That is why it is so important to stimulate the immune system and reduce inflammation of the cells. For this, food, exercise, and emotional balance play a crucial role.

As mentioned, food statistics in the Western world today show that 56 percent of our calories come from three sources:

1. refined sugar—fructose, cane sugar, corn syrup, etc.
2. white flour—white bread, white pasta, white rice, etc.
3. vegetable oils—soybean, sunflower, corn, etc.

These lack the vitamins, proteins, minerals, and omega-3 fatty acids that our bodies need for optimal functioning; in fact, they serve as food for cancer.

Sugar and white flour boost cellular inflammation and affect tumor growth. This has led many researchers to consider cancer as an epidemic due to the high amounts of insulin included in the daily intake. Obesity is also considered to be an epidemic.

It is critical to eat foods containing omega-3 and omega-6 fatty acids, which are known as essential because the human body does not produce them. Now, the amount of essential fatty acids will depend on what we eat, and, in turn, this will depend on what the cows and chickens we consume have eaten. If they are grass-fed, the meat, milk, and eggs will be in perfect balance between omega-3 and omega-6 (1:1). But if the animals eat corn and soy, we will be out of balance (1:15). That is why it's so important to eat organic meat, eggs, and dairy, although it is better not to eat this in excess.

Dietary Recommendations for Cancer Patients

- organic food—vegetables, fruit (all berries and green apples), raw nuts, whole-grain breads
- oatmeal—steel-cut
- wild-caught fish and salmon
- grass-fed meat
- green tea
- soy, miso, sprouts (great anti-cancer food)
- spices—tumeric (always adding black pepper) and curry
- mushrooms—shiitake, maitake, kawaratake, and enokitake
- dark chocolate (70 percent or more cacao)
- juicing
- ginger, garlic, onion
- brussel sprouts, cabbage, brocoli (steamed)
- raw honey
- alkaline water

It's also important to avoid GMOs, sugar, alcohol, iodized salt, and anything fried, unless you use coconut or avocado oil. Cook with avocado oil or flaxseed oil.

About Detoxifying

One of the causes of the sudden production of inflammatory substances implicit in the cellular functioning of every human being (and not mentioned much concerning cancer) is psychological stress. Every emotional outburst, every feeling of panic or anger causes the secretion of noradrenaline. (Noradrenaline is a neurotransmitter and a catecholamine-type hormone that is manufactured as a drug and produced naturally in the human body.) Like other neurotransmitters, the noradrenaline chemical triggers when the body needs to react quickly to a stressor; this neurotransmitter increases blood pressure and heart rate and gets the muscles ready to react. Unfortunately, these types of hormones are stimulants for cancerous tumors already present but dormant in our bodies.

Cancer is a disease with many edges, and there is much research about its origin. It's my intention that you, my friend, can see that it is not solely a physical problem. Many factors intervene; that is to say, bodies—the mental, the emotional, the physical (including physiology) and the spiritual bodies. All must be cared for to succeed in healing.

It's important to be aware of the food we eat to avoid ingesting foods that are not beneficial to our bodies. Detoxification in patients with cancer is crucial. We must help our bodies to release toxins so that they can function at an optimal level.

Some physicians, however, devote their time to patient care but are not always willing or able to investigate advances in medicine so they are updated in their field. Their treatment is based only on the information that the pharmaceutical industry offers them, which does not always mean it's ideal for each patient because each case is different. Representatives of the pharmaceutical industry visit doctors' offices to offer them the newest medications on the market. Some doctors may research the pharmaceutical supply, but others do not. As a matter of fact, there is so much research on cancer in so many parts of the world that it's hard to keep track of everything on the pharmaceutical market.

Natural methods also can be used to help patients, either in combination with drugs or other options within alternative medicine, such as acupuncture, homeopathy, or ayurveda. Natural options will *never* be opposed to any drug of artificial origin, and they will always act for health.

Everything that somehow does not benefit your body optimally will end up, sooner or later, being toxic in your system. Drug abuse suppresses the natural function of your body and creates resistance to medications; then it becomes necessary to increase dosages or to change the prescriptions. Meanwhile, your body is becoming contaminated, intoxicated, and, in some cases, limited in self-healing. The body loses its capacity to function innately.

You do not have to be sick to do a detox. This should be a habit in your life. Imagine that you have spent all the years of your life tossing your junk in a pond. After a while, it becomes infected or dries up. It's then necessary to clean it and to promote the flow of water currents to keep it clean.

If you are a person with constipation who does not drink at least two liters of water per day, who does not exercise, and who smokes, drinks alcohol, and eats junk food, surely your pond is polluted and rotten.

Understanding Detoxification and How to Detox

Lymphatic System

The lymphatic system consists of a set of fragile capillaries or ducts that spread throughout the body like a very dense spiderweb. They act in synchrony with the return or venous circulatory system. It helps the liquids, proteins, and molecular complexes that are trapped in tissues (because of difficulty in returning to the venous system) to be eliminated by other means. That is, the lymphatic fluid, when circulating, drags trapped substances and cleanses the tissues.

Lymphatic vessels are found throughout the body, except for the central nervous system, bone and cartilaginous tissue, and bone marrow. Lymph nodes provide antigens for purification fluids that contain everything from allergens to cancer cells. That fluid is called *lymph*.

Their capillaries are grouped and form large vessels that pour the lymph into the venous bloodstream. The lymph flows from the organs of the body to the heart and moves, thanks to a valve system that prevents its recoil.

Another important function of the lymphatic system is to manufacture antibodies or immunoglobulins for the immune system. Distributed throughout the network of lymphatic capillaries are the so-called lymph nodes. Their function is to contact defensive cells with the pathogens and/or antigens that circulate through the lymph, thus initiating the immune response.[3]

Lymph nodes usually become inflamed after a chemotherapy treatment and after being exposed to radiation. In my case, the doctors suggested taking a biopsy after my chemo treatment, as they "suspected" that my nodes were inflamed. Of course, they were inflamed because that happens regularly, but I decided to inform myself. My inner voice said that it was not a good idea to have a biopsy. After I investigated, I understood the behavior of the lymphatic system and knew that the biopsy would confirm the inflammation of my lymph nodes. The surgeons would not find what they were looking for, and then they would propose more surgeries. I declined flatly because my logic told me that it was not beneficial to expose my body to the stress of a surgery, even as "small" or "harmless" as it seemed. Also, no one could assure me that they wouldn't awaken or stimulate the sleeping monster (the tumor), which until then had been quiet. The physicians wanted to do a biopsy on my pleura too. I decided not to have any biopsies and instead to trust my intuition, to respect my body, and to avoid unnecessary invasive procedures.

The reason for my lymph inflammation was because my lymphatic system was working hard to produce white cells to fight the weakness of my immune system after the chemotherapy. Eventually, it would reduce to its normal size. It was just doing its natural job.

---

[3] JW Ball, JE Dains, JA Flynn, BS Solomon, and RW Stewart, "Lymphatic System," in *Seidel's Guide to Physical Examination* (Philadelphia, PA: Elsevier Mosby, 2015), [184-202].

After eighteen months, nothing bad had happened; on the contrary, my healing improved.

The goals of the lymphatic system us to

- feed the tissues,
- repair,
- manufacture, and
- participate in body defense mechanisms.

The main signs of intoxication in the body to watch out for are allergies, asthma, fatigue, unjustified tiredness, digestive problems, frequent infections, insomnia, skin problems, cellulite or obesity, and retention of liquids.

The lymphatic system is the sewer system for even common metabolic toxins and more so if there are health problems.

There is more lymph in the body than blood, but unlike blood, there is no pump for lymph. If the lymph is not moved from the small lymph nodes through the ducts into the kidneys and liver, the lymph will be clogged up, like a clogged drainage pipe. And the lack of exercise or movement of any kind is detrimental to lung and muscle health. The lymphatic system should be worked too.

1. Bouncing

Bouncing works very well to move lymphatic fluid enough for the kidneys and other organs of the body to purify. You can buy a mini-trampoline (about four feet in diameter) for about fifty dollars. It is advisable to bounce only for ten to fifteen minutes. You do not have to jump high, and you can hold on to something close to stabilize yourself if you have balance problems. Each time you bounce, you increase the force of gravity in your lymph.

With an intense walk or even a gentle bounce, the force of gravity is in vertical alignment with your body and your lymphatic system, thus causing a frictional force. You can also jump rope or jog, anything that serves to move the fluids of lymph nodes enough to facilitate the elimination of toxins. The exercise should be done outdoors in the most natural environment possible—with trees, next to a lake or the sea—at least twenty minutes a day or every other day.

Also, daily exercise promotes optimal breathing. We breathe automatically, but we often are not aware of what is involved in breathing or its benefits. When we breathe in, oxygen helps cleanse our blood. And when we exhale, we're excreting toxins that have been converted to CO_2. Yoga is a great exercise to practice breathing, in addition to stimulating the organs of the body.

Hydration is vital. Drink purified water often (two liters daily) to help the liver and kidneys to remove toxic lymphatic fluids from your body.

2.   The filters of the human body

So that the habitat of each cell is clean to receive oxygen and nutrients normally, the body has a cleaning service formed by the lymphatic system and five filters to discard the metabolic waste of the cells. These are as follows:

- The skin secretes uric acid, carbon dioxide, and cholesterol with sweat.
- The intestines excrete food residue through the stool.
- The lungs release carbon dioxide.
- The kidneys release uric acid through the urine.
- The liver secretes cholesterol through bile acids.
- The nutrients and useful substances are filtered and pass into the blood.

Of these five, three filter without stopping our blood; they are the lungs, the kidneys, and the liver. The pumping of the heart makes the blood circulate throughout the body. These three organs do not stop working while we are alive, and it is estimated that they can filter more than seven thousand liters of blood each day.

If the filters stop working, toxic waste accumulates in our bodies and invades cells, which die intoxicated or become cancerous. This transformation in carcinogens is the only thing that assures they will continue living in an intoxicated and very acidic environment.

Common wastes contaminate our bodies. These are cause, for example, by

- drinking alcohol or soft drinks,
- using toxic cleaning products, which are the majority,
- eating lots of meat and few raw and fresh foods,
- eating refined products, such as sugar, flour, and salt,
- breathing polluted air, like tobacco smoke or car exhaust,
- consuming aggressive drugs or pharmacological treatment,
- exposure to preservatives and pesticides in food, and/or
- the malfunction of a purifying organ.[4]

3. Coffee enemas

The purpose of the enema is to remove toxins accumulated in the liver and to remove free radicals from the bloodstream. The caffeine travels via the hemorrhoidal vein and the portal system to the liver, opens up the bile ducts, and allows the liver to release bile, which contains toxins.

Coffee administered rectally also stimulates an enzyme system in the liver called glutathione S-transferase by 600–700 percent above normal activity levels. This enzyme reacts with free radicals (which cause cell damage) in the bloodstream and makes them inert.

The patient holds the coffee enema in the colon for twelve to fifteen minutes. During this time, the body's entire blood supply passes through the liver four to five times, carrying poisons picked up from the tissues. The enema acts as a form of dialysis of the blood across the gut wall.

---

[4] https://www.naturopatamasdeu.com/la-importancia-limpiar-los-filtros-de-nuestro-cuerpo.

The purpose of the coffee enema is not to clear out the intestines, but the quart of water in the enema stimulates peristalsis in the gut. A portion of the water also dilutes the bile and increases the bile flow, thereby flushing toxic bile (loaded with toxins by the glutathione S-transferase enzyme system) out of the intestines.

Additionally, coffee enemas can help to relieve pain, nausea, general nervous tension, and depression.[5]

4. Radiation

Radiation is odorless, colorless, and tasteless. We can't easily avoid exposure to this environmental contaminant. There is an abundance of research to confirm that electronic devices are radioactive contamination, and they deliver far more radiation than is commonly believed, especially scans that give off ionizing radiation. In a lot of cases, the benefits from medical scans, when needed, do outweigh the initial threat of cancer from radiation. However, while this is true, it is also important to realize that our DNA could be damaged. The body's cells will attempt to repair themselves, but many times, they replicate damaged or unhealthy cells. This can lead to DNA mutations and potentially contribute to cancer down the road. Our bodies can sometimes be bombarded by different types of radiation that weaken the body's cells. It's not our fault, and most of it we cannot control.[6]

Common sources of environmental radiation exposure are as follows:

- x-rays/mammograms
- CT scans
- PET scans
- other types of imaging tests or scans that emit radiation

---

[5] "A Cancer Therapy: Results of Fifty Cases by Dr. Gerson," *Healing the Gerson Way* by Charlotte Gerson, and *Liver Detoxification with Coffee Enemas* by Morton Walker, DPM, excerpted from July 2001 edition of *Townsend Newsletter*.
[6] http://www.radiexposure.com.

- airport security scanners/airplane travel
- electronics/communications equipment—cell phones, computers, wireless devices
- electromagnetic fields (EMFs)
- geopathic stress
- nuclear radiation/fallout from nuclear disasters, such as Fukushima
- fallout from atmospheric testing of nuclear weapons in the 1940s, 1950s, 1960s, and 2000s.[7]

5. Fasting

Recent studies at the University of California, Berkeley, stated that three-day water fasts reset the immune system by activating the stem cells and enabling us to perform at the optimum level. Three to four days of water fasting is good for detoxifying your body. This will help clean out your system.

Another simpler way than doing a full water fast is intermittent fasting. Begin with a twelve-hour fast, then twenty-four hours, and then a forty-eight-hour fast. Essentially, within a week you do not eat anything for one day, and this will allow the liver and kidneys to detoxify completely and get rid of all the toxins. It is, however, important to hydrate yourself within that twenty-four-hour span with lots of water. Some people like to do a twenty-one-day fast.

6. Infrared sauna

Sweating is your body's natural way of purging itself to maintain a healthy state. The human body has millions of microscopic sweat glands that are infused with fluid, brought there by the bloodstream. These glands empty that fluid to the skin's surface as a cooling mechanism when the body overheats, flushing out any toxins and heavy metals carried there.

---

[7] Ibid.

Infrared sauna wavelengths reduce the size of water clumps in the body, invigorate them, and help them to combine with toxins. Decreasing the size of the water clumps and letting them vibrate allows them to propel out of cells and body tissue, taking with them toxins that were previously held inside. These toxins are removed from the body by the urine and feces, breath, and through the skin.

The purpose of any infrared sauna is to make the body to sweat over an extended period (fifteen to thirty minutes), carrying with it plenty of toxins due to a raised core body temperature.

7. Epsom salt detox bath

An Epsom salt detox bath is an extraordinary external way to detox and gets out any unhealthy and artificial substances. Skin is the largest organ of the body and the main detox medium of our bodies; therefore, it's a great detoxifying method.

A detox bath stimulates the lymph system and promotes increments of oxygen and blood flow to the body. This kind of bath helps reinforce the immune system and soothes the body. The sulfates from Epsom salts are benficial, as they are necessary for the formation of proteins in the digestive tract. Sulfates also motivate the pancreas to form digestive enzymes that are necessary to detoxify the body. This detox bath will help remove toxins and support in defending the body from heavy metals. Soaking in Epsom salts also raises the body's magnesium levels, as it is easily absorbed.

The normal amount to use is two cups of Epsom salts for a regular-size bathtub. If your bathtub is larger or smaller, you may want to modify the amount. It is most helpful to soak in the bathtub for thirty to forty minutes. That allows enough time for your body to exclude the toxins and to assimilate minerals in the water.

Essential oils such as lavender, lemon, sandalwood, cilantro, or melaleuca will help in obtaining therapeutic benefits and support in the detoxification process.

These are some of the ways to help our bodies eliminate toxins. You can make use one of them, some of them, or all of them. You'll know which one suits you best. Make your decision based on whatever your body demands of you; that is, follow your intuition.

Listen to Your Body

Many people do not know that the body speaks to us and sometimes yells when it is not heard. Do you remember any occasion when you heard your body? What did your body tell you? Are you connected to your body?

Throughout my professional practice, I have seen patients with many different diagnoses. Their bodies, indeed, had given them warnings, but they didn't pay attention. Maybe they were very busy, or they were conflicted by what they heard. Maybe they were afraid or had no idea what to do.

For many years, I heard my body, but I didn't listen because I was busy taking care of my family and patients. Also, I did not like what my body was saying to me, and I simply turned the page so I woudln't have to deal with those issues that my body insisted on reminding me.

Here are just a few examples of what my body was saying:

- Sleep the necessary hours.
- Eat at the indicated times.
- Give yourself time to rest and have some inner peace.
- Revisit your childhood wounds that you have not solved yet.
- Laugh more often.
- Stop searching for perfection.
- You are demanding too much of yourself.

My body yelled at me for months, until one day, I had a car accident. Fortunately, nothing serious happened, but before long, I developed a cough. In the beginning, I thought it was because of the accident. Then I thought it was because of an allergy, but when I went out of town, my cough continued. It became clear that it was not an allergy, as I was no longer exposed to the environment that I thought was causing the allergy. I decided to go to the pulmonologist, and there began the *via crusis*.

I assumed that my body would take the pressure, as many people do. We take our bodies for granted. We are not aware that the body is sacred; it is a temple, and therefore we must respect and honor it and give it the care it deserves.

I have never been addicted to cigarrettes, alcohol, or drugs. I have always taken care of the quality of the food I eat. But the level of stress with which I lived was too much. I juggled my family and my work, and that caused me too much stress. I did not know how to say no or how to establish healthy limits. Stress had been in my life since an early age; I now realize that despite having what might be considered a normal childhood, I lived with a lot of stress. It was the same when I was a teenager, which already is a tense transition stage.

For about two or three years before my diagnosis, my body was telling me that I needed a liver detox. I never did it. I began to lose hair, but I thought it was because of stress or some problem with food. *Maybe I have a vitamin deficiency,* I thought. Deep down, though, a voice said, *What if it's cancer?* Many times I heard my body say to me, *Get an MRI of the whole body.* But in thinking about what it would cost and the fear that my voice might be right, I simply nullified that calling. I was convinced that the voice was a paranoid voice and not the wisdom of my body that was warning me.

Your body, soul, and mind are meant to be in unity. To guarantee that they are, your entire being is based on feedback links. Mind, body, and soul are related, though sometimes they take turns in leading. They are not three different elements of our beings. Consciousness is the connection. It is crucial to be aware of who is leading (Body? Mind? Soul?) in order to have positive outlets for your health. Every cell recognizes when you are sad, anxious, or stressed. A cell's attentiveness is expressed in chemical reactions. The message comes through loud and clear. Our thoughts stimulate a symptom in our bodies, and a symptom is a manifestation of our thoughts and, therefore, of our reality.

How can we learn to listen to our bodies? We don't need to learn because it's already an innate skill. The following ideas, however, will help you recognize, accept, and listen to the voice of your body:

- In Buddhist philosophy, there is much talk of impermanence, which means that nothing is permanent; everything changes. Therefore, we are constantly changing. From one moment to another, our mood can change. We age from day to day, but at the same time, we regenerate. I recommend that you accept those changes and be open to them. Flow with impermanence.
- Be willing to listen to your body. It's always speaking, so set aside the fear.
- Don't deny what you feel; accept it without judgment.
- Trust the wisdom of your cells. Actually, you are a sack of hundreds of billions of partners.
- Give your body what it wants to do: rest, be active, eat different types of food.

Have you eaten something that upset your body? How do you know it affected you? Your body tells you, perhaps through dermatitis, or inflammation of the colon, or sometimes through diarrhea. That is communication between the body and you, but if you do not listen, you might eat again whatever caused those symptoms in your body.

There is a great deal of literature regarding the hidden messages in each organ of the body that manifest as a symptom or illness. For example, the stomach is related to anger; lungs to sadness; and the uterus to issues related to family (home). The skeletal system represents our structure, and the throat is related to expression (what is said and not said).[8] These are examples of how to listen to your body and how to understand each organ's relationship with the root of discomfort. Through inquiry, we can reach a deep communication, and with a good direction, we can even heal the illness.

---

[8] Eric Rolf, *La medicina del Alma* (Madrid, España: Ediciones Gaia, 2003).

Questions for Reflection

- What type of diet do you have?
- What type of cravings do you have?
- Do you feel that your environment is toxic (at work or at home)?
- Do you practice any method of detox?
- Do you have an exercise routine?
- Do you listen to your body? How frequently?

Chapter 4

THE RELATIONSHIP BETWEEN YOUR EMOTIONS AND YOUR BODY

Had I left images hidden in the emotions, I might have been torn to pieces by them.
—Carl Jung

The Triad of Being: Mind, Body and Spirit

Have you ever had a sore throat? Have you ever been unable to speak after a situation in which you were insulted or humiliated? Did you ever feel as if you had a knot in your throat? How many times do we want to respond to a comment or an insult, but we keep quiet to avoid further consequences?

Have you had a stomachache or colitis? Or maybe you've had the feeling that something is stuck in the stomach. Have you been nauseated? How many times have you wanted to "vomit" a situation? Think how your emotions make instant changes in your physique. When you're too anxious or stressed, do you get a headache? Do you have an allergy or sinus issue without a specific cause? With a little self-awareness, we can perceive that our bodies reflect our emotions, mainly those that we suppress.

Psychosomatics is an area in medicine that studies mind-body relation. Psychic factors can impact physical disorders, which are used by medical professionals and psychologists to understand the origin of some diseases. These include hereditary, genetic, and environmental factors, but their damage may increase as a result of psychic stress; the emotional state can often determine the course of the illness.

Some health professionals, unfortunately, seek only to understand the disease and not the person as a whole. They completely disregard the human being as a totality and resort to palliatives that distract the finding of the cause, which makes the remission of the disease more difficult. Often the patients prefer a drug as a substitute for psychotherapy or another resource that will help them work their psyches. Many consider medication to be the best solution and perhaps the easiest, and most people want quick solutions. In many cases, the medication is essential, but it does not always eliminate the causes, as it's only a palliative that relieves the symptoms. There may be psychological issues behind the physical ills that afflict us.

Repressing feelings is a significant cause of ills in the body; in other words, sicknesses arise and are worsened by the difficulty of expressing our feelings, as we manifest in the body what we cannot solve in the psyche. The factor that leads to the worsening of diseases is a drop in immunity because the emotions first reach the immune system. When we face a struggle, we may suffer from flu symptoms or allergies, which arise when our immunity is low. That is, any organic disorder is related to the emotional state, conscious or unconscious, recent or not.

We think we have solved a problem that afflicts us, but in reality, we have only buried it; it's placed in different parts of the body— bitterness, resentment, anger, frustrations—that over the years add up. Not thinking about something that hurt us doesn't mean it no longer hurts us; it simply may be suppressed in our subconscious.

The body is like a screen where the emotions are projected, and negative emotions are projected as diseases. Such somatizations occur in the short or long term, as each mind and body respond according to its own time, and all the negative feelings that we repress can give rise to illnesses if we keep them for a long time. That is why we must resolve the questions that trouble us—everything that bothers us—therefore limiting our subconscious from talking through the language of the body. The psychic factor predominates and is the origin of almost all diseases throughout life.

In recent years, it has been scientifically proven that psychological stress affects the immune system, weakening the body's natural defenses and making it more vulnerable to assaults of all kinds. *Psychoneuroimmunology*, a new field of medical research, studies the relation of the mind to the defenses of the body; namely, the way in which thoughts act on the cells. One of the findings is that the brain hormone ACTH flows into the blood during stressful situations, slows the action of lymphocytes (a type of white blood cell, leukocyte, that is of fundamental importance in the immune system[9]), and inhibits their ability to generate antibodies. The hypothalamus transmits chemical and electrical messages to the pituitary gland, which in turn sends the hormone ACTH to the adrenal glands, which activates a series of chemical messengers. One of them is cortisol, which modifies the action of lymphocytes and also has a great influence on our propensity to contract serious diseases, like cancer, for instance.

Eric Rolf is a Western spiritually based teacher and counselor. He was born in New York City in 1936 and has dedicated his life to the exploration of the creative and communication processes from their inner sources. He is also well known for his natural self-healing and personal self-realization activities with both individuals and groups of all types.

Within his practice, he began to notice surprising changes in the results of his consultations and also in his own body. He noticed common characteristics among people who suffered the same type of physical problem and their ways of seeing life. This was how he established a relationship between a psychological problem and physical illness.

Other specialists also have observed this phenomenon. Is it a coincidence that patients with similar symptoms have similar histories? The common response has been that everyone creates

---

[9] https://www.britannica.com/science/lymphocyte.

their own reality. (In chapter 5, I will mention other specialists who have come to the same conclusions as Rolf.)

There is a third ingredient in this formula: the soul, which it is expressed continuously. We're not always aware of its expression, but it still exists. We may believe that what happens outside is alien to us, instead of realizing that it is actually the manifestation of our interior. The soul guides us to live a series of necessary experiences, and if we don't live in fullness, it can trigger a specific health problem.

Body Language

Body language is not generally explored in everyday life because we aren't aware of it. Nevertheless, it is the axis and the remedy of many psychological problems. Most people are victims of the tension produced by their environments, and, as I've mentioned, that environment is often a response to a reality that they build from recurrent thoughts. In spite of this, the body, in its struggle for survival, can lose its sensibility. There is a nullification of the body. Alexander Lowen, a pioneer in the field of bioenergetic analysis, demonstrates cleverly that the body is the mirror of the personality and is the place where emotional disorders manifest themselves.

During my process with cancer, I was convinced that I should address the cancer from all possible fronts. One of the first therapies I took was psycho-corporal therapy (from the bioenergetic approach). It was a confrontational experience. My therapist exposed me to a series of physical exercises in which I made body awareness of a series of emotions contained in my body, even though my mind wasn't aware of them. The extensive literature on this subject ensures that the lungs are related to sadness, melancholy, and fear of death, among other emotions. I did not relate to these emotions because my life seemed to have more joy than sadness. As a result of my psycho-corporal therapies, I had the revelation of the clear and surprising relationships that exist between the functioning of myself and my personal history, as well as the patterns of my body movements (posture) and my muscular tensions.

Thus, I discovered the configuration of my person, disturbed under several layers, anchored in the tension and anxiety of my reality, and sustained in a past of events that marked me unconsciously.

The lungs are the border that separates our inner world from the outer world. It defines boundaries and protects perimeters. The lungs defend the organism from the aggressions of pathogens, preventing the disease installed in our bodies. Well-toned lungs will give us a sense of strength and endurance against adversity.

The lungs are related to the survival instinct. In my therapeutic process, I became aware that for many years, I felt invaded (I'd allowed it) and did not know how to establish healthy and firm boundaries in some interpersonal relationships or at moments that were toxic to me. When the lungs function correctly, we instinctively and spontaneously capture situations of danger and know how to react properly. At some point in my life, however, my lungs lost the energy to exert this protective function.

In this case of imbalance, it made me vulnerable, and I felt unsafe. I somehow lost the instinct for survival so that I perceived melancholy and abandonment, when, in fact, I was characterized as being extroverted and cheerful.

As mentioned, the emotion related to the lungs is sadness. Sadness seized me without my realizing what I tended to isolate, to the point that I became paralyzed and desensitized to my own emotions to avoid being hurt.

When I understood this, I realized it from the body—that is, my body reacted to this consciousness—not from the mind, as the corporal exercise led me to this magically. This was a healing moment because I had reached a point of balance and a mental, corporal, and spiritual connection.

Dr. Hamer and New German Medicine

In August 1978, Ryke Geerd Hamer, MD, at that time chief of internists at the oncology clinic at the University of Munich, Germany, received the terrible news that his only son had been shot. He died in December 1978. A few months later, Dr. Hamer was diagnosed with testicular cancer. Since he had never been seriously ill, he immediately assumed that this development of cancer could be directly related to the tragic loss of his son.

The death of his son and his own experience with cancer motivated Dr. Hamer to investigate the personal history of his cancer patients. He immediately learned that, just as he had, all his patients had gone through some unusually stressful episode before they developed cancer. The observation of a mind-body connection was not surprising. Numerous studies had already taught that a traumatic event often precedes cancer and other diseases.

But Dr. Hamer's research gained importance when he sought to hypothesize that all bodily events are controlled from the brain. He analyzed his patients' brain scans and compared them with his medical records. Dr. Hamer discovered that every disease—not just cancer—is controlled from its own specific area of the brain and linked to a very particular and identifiable *conflict clash*.

The result of his research is a scientific precedent that illustrates the biological relationship between the psyche and the brain in correlation with the organs and tissues of the entire human body.

Dr. Hamer called his discoveries the Five Laws of New Medicine. These biological laws, which apply to any patient case, offer a new understanding of the cause, development, and natural healing process of diseases.

Dr. Hamer suffered rejection from the medical community in Germany and was asked to give up his findings, as well as being denied the renewal of his professional license. He was persecuted and harassed for almost thirty years, particularly by the German and French authorities.

In 1997, Dr. Hamer moved to Spain, where he lived in exile until his death on July 2, 2017 (during the process of my writing this book). He had continued his research and fought for the official recognition of his New Medicine until his last breath.[10]

I had known and read about Dr. Hamer for many years, so as soon as I received my diagnosis, I wanted to know what had triggered my cancer, just as he had, since I have no family history of cancer. I reviewed my family tree, and I went to a couple of bio-decoding sessions, several psycho-corporal therapies, and a few Family Constellations sessions. That's how I got to the point of assimilating the event that programmed cancer and the one that detonated it. I was able to get to the biological origin of my cancer, and therefore, I had the opportunity to continue working on that topic from other perspectives to help me deepen, tear off, and heal the root. Art journaling has undoubtedly been an extremely useful tool for shaping my thoughts and emotions, and it has also been a thread in my entire process from the beginning. (I will discuss this technique in chapter 7.)

Bio-decoding

Bio-decoding is a methodology that seeks to deactivate or neutralize the emotional factors, or programs, that led to a symptom, pain, illness, or allergy and that trigger a malaise. Bio-decoding allows us to find out through the symptoms, which may be the emotional origin of the disease. It is a methodology based on the biological meaning of symptoms or illness.

Christian Fleche—born in France and considered the father of the biological decoding of diseases and founder of the French School of Bio-decoding (*Décodage Biologique*)—explains that this methodology seeks the coherence of the symptom.

The goal of this technique is to look for the codes that connect a symptom with a specific emotion. By working that emotion, we

---

[10] Summary of the New Medicine, Dr. Ryke Geerd Hamer.

can reach better mental or behavioral states that then are reflected in the state of health.

This methodology can be applied to the emotions that are experienced in acute, chronic, and cancerous diseases; organic dysfunctions; insomnia; eating disorders; fertility problems; muscle or joint pain; fibromyalgia; allergies; compulsions; addictions; phobias; stress; anxiety; and depression, among others.

Having said this, this way of approaching the disease is crucial also because it is a way to find the emotional root of the disease from the biological point of view. There could have been a situation in which the body received a bio-shock, where this specific event generated an emotion; then that emotion was imprinted on the cells in such a way that it detonated as a disease that was already programmed beforehand.

In the past eight years, I have witnessed bio-decoding sessions led by a leading therapist in México, who, as it turned out, is my former psychoanalyst. I have witnessed the effectiveness of this methodology, in which the patients discover the hidden message (or code) of their diseases. I saw patients with fibromyalgia reach the emotional origin that paralyzed them, which years later manifested as fibromyalgia. I saw patients with cancer experience the moment when they imprinted an emotion on their cells, which, years later, their bodies manifested as cancer. Having witnessed this so many times, I understood that it was time for me to face the imprinted ghost in my cells, to find the emotion that programmed cancer and the event that detonated it.

It was certainly a confrontational and powerful experience, but at the same time, it was releasing. Like the vast majority of cases, mine was related to my family history and my way of assimilating that story with mine. There was an aha moment. It is not with the purpose of returning to the past and being victimized; the goal is to raise awareness of the fact.

In Lewis Carroll's *Alice's Adventures in Wonderland*, Alice says, "It's no use going back to yesterday because I was a different person then." True! Buddhists talk about impermanence, yet taking a look at the family or personal history can be beneficial in freeing ourselves from the burden of the collective family unconsciousness.

Family Constellations

Why is it important to go back to our genealogy tree? In its beginning, psychoanalysis affirmed that the psychic life of any individual was sustained in the relationship with his/her family, especially with the parents. Sigmund Freud argued that the nature of the bonds between parents and children in early childhood were decisive for their adult personalities. The origin of the neurosis was fundamentally in the repressed drives in that first stage of the life. Carl Jung went further and supported the existence of what he called the "collective unconscious." In fact, he studied his own genealogical tree in depth.[11][12]

Systemic psychology and the tool of the Family Constellations technique constitute methods widely used in family psychotherapy of our times. Systemic therapy has provided valuable insight into the influence of the family on the psyche and each individual's way of acting in the world.[13]

Understanding the nature of our family trees and our relationships and discovering our family's unconscious patterns reveal the dynamics that carry identifications and implications from one generation to the next, which can make our lives difficult. Working in our own roots is a healing process in the sense that it opens us to the opportunity to see the dynamics from another perspective. When we are young, we learn the history of our country and our culture, but we often don't pay attention to our family history, which marks us for good or for bad.

---

[11] Constelaciones, Abrazos y Acuerdos… Familiares, Otra mirada al pasado para seguir adelante. Rosa Döring Hermosillo.

[12] "Constelaciones Familiares": Fundamentación sistémica de Bert Hellinger; Mónica Giraldo Perez, Carmen Cecilia Vargas Sierra.

[13] Ibid.

I heard about the Family Constellations technique about twenty years ago. The first time I attended a workshop, I didn't know what to expect, but I trusted the facilitator, whom I'd known since I was seven years old. (She had been my psychoanalyst.) It was fascinating to discover and solve issues of my family that I had not consciously realized were affecting me in my daily life. I started to host more workshops with my former psychoanalyst, and I continued to participate in countless Family Constellations, directly or indirectly. I learned a lot from all of them. I managed to put my family tree in order, which helped me to find answers and to be aware of patterns and burdens that I did not want to continue transmitting to my children and future generations in my tribe.

Connecting with Your Emotions

When we become aware of the presence of an emotion and identify it, we are not only in the here and now, but we are honest with ourselves. A mind disconnected from the body can be a source of suffering and ignorance.

Emotional intelligence is the ability to perceive one's own emotions and those of others, thus promoting empathy. Becoming aware means identifying and properly recognizing our own experience, which then helps us to understand each other better. When we recognize the emotion, we can work on what has caused that emotion, as well as being able to handle it.

Usually, the first emotion shown is anger. It is like a porcupine, which, when it feels threatened, shows its thorns to defend itself. As humans, when we are afraid or feel attacked or in danger, we show anger instinctively to avoid being hurt. But underneath anger, there is fear, sadness, frustration, and so on. Anger is manifested as a defense mechanism.

Emotion reveals itself to an inner or outer situation. That is, our own thoughts may be triggering an emotion, or an external fact may trigger another emotion. The important thing is to become aware of which emotion we feel, as well as from what or who.

To the extent that we connect with our own emotions and become aware of the origin, we can be more responsible for our behavior. Many times I ask my patients if they know what emotion they feel and in what part of their bodies they feel it. In many cases, this makes them aware of the relationship of their emotion with their illness or pain, if any, or their relation to recurring health problems, since each damaged organ responds to a feeling.

Emotions give flavor to life. The key is to find the emotion blocked to achieve a joyous life.

> *Illness is the effort that Nature makes to heal the mankind.*
> —Carl G. Jung

From my experience, understanding the following emotions is essential to set free and heal from that which hurts or keeps us stuck. I present them in the order in which they must be addressed:

1. Forgiveness

To speak of emotions is to speak of fear, melancholy, shame, anger, joy, resignation, tenderness, empathy, repentance, envy, indignation, panic, jealousy, loneliness, surprise, and humiliation, among others. We can have positive or negative emotions, but negative emotions likely will generate resentment. If nothing is done about it, such resentment begins to weigh on our bodies. And this is where forgiveness has to appear on the scene.

Sometimes the word *forgiveness* is associated with a religious theme, but is beyond that; it's about the spiritual realm. Some may think that forgiving has to do with tolerance of those who offend us, and then forgiving is a way to nullify our feelings. To forgive, however, is not to justify who did us harm. Forgiveness is an inner work of emotional liberation. Regardless of who has offended or aggrieved you, the act of forgiveness does not require you to see yourself face-to-face with that person.

Nevertheless, ego is skillful and will do the impossible so that you do not go through the process of forgiveness. As long as you are clear that you may forgive others—not because they deserve it, but because you deserve the inner peace—that will give the release of such resentment.

Cancer (or any disease) is a bundle of emotions that change day by day; sometimes we experience several emotions on the same day. And if we do not do any internal work of recognition of the forgiveness, it is difficult to advance in healing. It is as if every emotion that was retained or denied was a burden.

Forgiveness—genuine forgiveness from the heart—is the most effective way to free yourself from the internal negativity that will help you to live in the inner peace you deserve and that corresponds to you by divine right. Although it is not easy to quiet the ego, it is not impossible. The clue is to find the balance between ego and forgiveness. Meditation is a great tool to achieve this balance. Quiet the mind and feel the heart, thus achieving coherence between the two.

As Jack Kornfield mentions in his book *The Wise Heart*[14], "Like the practice of compassion, forgiveness does not ignore the truth of our suffering." Forgiveness is not weakness; it demands courage and integrity. Yet only forgiveness and love can bring about the peace we long for.

Forgiveness is fundamentally for our own sake, for our own mental health. It is a way to let go of the pain we carry.

2. Vulnerability

Talking about cancer is talking about vulnerability. Culturally, vulnerability is associated with weakness, but from my point of view, it is an act that demands a lot of courage. Sometimes, it is not easy

---

[14] Kornfield, Jack. *The Wise Heart: A Guide to the Universal Teachings of Buddhist Psychology*. Bantam Dell, 2008.

to accept being vulnerable (at least not for me), much less showing yourself as vulnerable to the world.

The first months after my diagnosis of cancer, I decided to withdraw myself for few months. First, it was because the news had a great impact on my biology and psyche; second, because I needed to isolate myself to avoid the external noise and to focus on the decisions I had to make, as literally, it was a matter of life or death. I also needed silence so I could hear my inner voice and know which steps to take in my healing process. Another reason I isolated myself was an instinct for self-protection.

The word *cancer* has a connotation of death, so my instinct told me that my attitude needed to be 100 percent positive and to avoid exposure to negative, insensitive, or inopportune comments and people.

When people know that someone is dealing with cancer, they are not always the most helpful. That's not because they are bad or mean people, but it's not easy to know what to say to the person who is going through a health challenge of this magnitude. Therefore, I decided to avoid those comments, mostly because I felt vulnerable. I think I instinctively sought refuge.

But over time, I had another type of vulnerability; it was like climbing a mountain. At first, the mountain seems unconquerable, but little by little, you gain ground, until again, it is difficult to take the road up. Each break on the way to the top of the mountain represents a moment of vulnerability and uncertainty.

I had moments of such vulnerability, and I still have them because vulnerability is a way of stripping the soul, of showing myself to the rest of the world—without filters, without cover, without shields. And those moments also are moments of lucidity, of liberation of acceptance, of creativity, enlightenment, and strength.

Imagine that you are on a very high bridge. You're attached to a rubber band, about to jump into the void, and you only can trust the rubber band will sustain you. There is no going backward. In this process, I had to jump several times from the bridge, releasing control and trusting and having faith in God/universe. I know He always has my back.

Vulnerability can be defined as the diminished capacity of a person or a group of people to anticipate, cope, and resist the effects of a natural hazard or one caused by human activity, and to recover from them. Vulnerability is almost always associated with poverty, but people living in isolation, insecurity, and defenselessness in the face of risks, traumas, or pressures are also vulnerable.

The other side of the coin is capacity, which can be described as the resources available to individuals, families, and communities to deal with a threat or to resist the effects of a hazard. These resources can be physical or material, but they can also be found in the way a community is organized or in the skills or attributes of the people and/or organizations of the community.

Now, surely vulnerability is key to continuing evolution and learning in life. Vulnerability can occur in many life situations, but in order to fulfill the objective of vulnerability, it is necessary to soak in it. You need to step on the ground in order to push outward and be covered with the courage required to get ahead of any challenge; in other words, to surrender. If the vulnerability is reversed, if it avoids, it will not have fulfilled its mission. The affected person probably will not have an evolution in his or her existence, which is not serious; perhaps it's not what they had to learn in this lifetime.

Within my healing process, there were two moments of extreme vulnerability. One was at the very moment of the diagnosis of lung cancer. This feeling of vulnerability lasted for about two months, until one of the doctors said that I had to remove my left lung. That's when I went from vulnerability to courage—courage to take the reins of my life and my health, to be responsible for myself.

The second time I had an appointment with vulnerability—and these meetings were unpredictable; I never knew when it would occur—was when I returned to the clinic to continue with my IPT treatment. One week after this treatment, my hair began to fall out in piles. It was like losing layers that somehow protected me from seeing myself as sick, to disguise an indisputable reality. I've had long hair since I was a girl. I used to play with it doing different hairstyles. Also, in general, hair frames the face, especially for women. It is a symbol, to a certain extent, of sensuality and can be an element of vanity.

One day I was in front of the mirror with a brush in my hand, holding a mountain of hair, and I decided it was inevitable that I would shave my head. It was a confrontational moment; it was a test of reality. I cried. I felt vulnerable. I sensed that I was losing a significant part of myself. Something that represented (in my view) what I was. How could I let it go? How could I show myself in front of the mirror and to the world so raw?

At that moment, my husband came into the bathroom, and I told him that I had decided to shave my head. With tears in our eyes, he hugged me. It was not a simple hug; it was a container hug, a compassionate hug full of love. And in that love, we fused the two of us in silence and passed from pain to courage; to the strength and determination that a situation like this gives you. In the end, I said, "It's just hair. It will grow. Renew or die!"

At first, it wasn't easy to go out with a scarf on my head, but soon, it became fun to use scarves and combine them with my clothes. To my surprise, many people told me, "That's definitely your look," and I don't think they said it to cheer me up. I felt excellent about the new *raw* Valentina. It gave a new perspective to my being. People who didn't know about my healing process never questioned whether the scarf was covering my baldness.

3.   Resilience

Each person has an innate self-regulation tendency, which means a capacity for resilience. And this ability is related to one's true spiritual being, as perceived beyond several spiritual traditions and thinkers.

Some people may remain calm in the face of disaster or life challenges, while others don't. But this is due to the ability to cope with problems and difficulties. These difficulties may be related to financial issues, illness, natural disasters, loss, and so on. Instead of falling into despair or avoiding the situation, resilient people face the adversity by using their skills and strength. We all are resilient, but some people find a way to accept their vulnerability with grace, to surrender, to have introspection of the situation with courage, and then move on.

But if we are stuck with ego's power, if we instead have self-pity, if we insist on play the role of victim, then the challenges will persist over and over until we understand the meaning of resilience in our lives. Ego will always try to convince us to judge (self-judgment and others) and will look for a way to confuse us, like the siren's song, to avoid listening to our intuition and our truth. Those who allow their inner voices to speak are the ones who practice resilience.

Here's an example: Imagine that you're holding a dry, square sponge, and you soak it in a container of water. Then you squeeze the sponge until it's almost dry. It will lose its shape for a moment, but it will recover its original form in seconds. That is how we respond to challenges; they come into our lives and compress our souls, but after a time, we can recover our size and shape. But we need to surrender, to let go of control in order to allow the situation to reshape us and to achieve growth. Humility is an indispensable ingredient if you want to become a healthy, resilient person.

4.   Gratitude

Once we genuinely forgive, we accept vulnerability and courage. Once we surrender and humbly understand our resilience, then we can feel the transforming power of gratitude.

The first time I heard about gratitude as an emotion was in a TED Talk that I saw on YouTube. I was so impressed and excited by Louie Schwartzberg's lecture, images, and passion that I was in love with his work. Schwartzberg is an award-winning cinematographer, director, and producer who captures breathtaking images and stories that celebrate life. From then on, I decided to lead gratitude workshops to offer people the opportunity to connect to this emotion.

But it was not until I had the cancer diagnosis and worked through my emotions that I truly understood the power of gratitude. Louie bases his work on the beauty of nature. I think that's what got me hooked. I always take pictures of the sky, bugs, flowers, trees, and so on. I firmly believe that a sense of awe and wonder is necessary because it makes us feel alive and part of nature as it soothes the spirit. I have always been amazed by nature's beauty, but I did not make the connection with gratitude until I saw Schwartzberg's artwork.

He said,

> Beauty and seduction are nature's tools for survival because we protect what we fall in love with; it opens our heart and make us realize that we are part of nature and we are not separate from it. When we see ourselves in nature, it also connects us to every one of us because is clear that is all connected in one[15].

Through his images, he awakens the feeling of gratitude—the gratitude of being able to sense the beauty that surrounds us.

Here's another example: imagine you are buried under layers of emotions—anger, despair, resentment, abandonment—and you're unable to see or breathe through these layers. Everything is dark in your surroundings. But as you forgive, as you allow yourself to be vulnerable, as you connect with your resilience ability, then you can remove the heavy layers that have blinded and begin to blossom. The light starts to appear, and the air begins to circulate in such a way that you can live lightly and live your life with gratitude. Now you can see everything through the eyes of appreciation. That's when you can feel and vibrate in harmony with yourself and with everything around you. It is when you understand the value of the here and now—the generous present moment. It's when you value every moment of your life and each being that surrounds you.

---

[15] https://www.youtube.com/watch?v=-aEhSgyWZe0

This emotion lasts as long as you choose. Life keeps happening, but that does not imply that you disconnect from it. That's why the power of gratitude is transformative. You begin to live your life in a compassionate state—self-compassion and compassion for others.

When I have a feeling of gratitude, my eyes fill with tears—I can't help myself. Those moments are pure fullness. I just close my eyes and give thanks to God and the universe for that very moment.

Questions for Reflection

- Did you find a relationship between your illness and your family story?
- Did you find a relationship between your illness and your personal story?
- Have you forgiven yourself for the harm you have done to yourself (unconsciously and conciously)? Have you forgiven others?
- What is a situation or situations when you felt vulnerable?
- Has there been any challenge where you encountered resilience?
- Do you recognize how it feels to be grateful?
- What are you grateful for?

Chapter 5

THE POWER OF YOUR THOUGHTS

Your thoughts are incredibly powerful. Choose yours wisely.
—Dr. Joe Dispenza

The Brain and the Mind

Almost everything we know about the brain is based on its physiological functioning. It's the central organ of the central nervous system. Among the physical aspects of the brain, we know of all those related to a biological point of view, which can be reduced to physical and chemical terms; for example, the anatomical, physiological, biochemical, biophysical, and embryological points of view.

The brain is one of the most complex and mysterious organs in the body. It is so complex that today, we know only a small part of the brain's operation and its capabilities, despite huge steps in neuroscience.

In recent years, however, significant research and discoveries have been made about the brain and its neuroplasticity, and this has increased our knowledge about this vital organ. The study of the human brain has been carried out from different points of view in various disciplines and at different levels. These studies could roughly be divided into two main aspects: the physical aspect and the mental aspect. On the other hand, all the knowledge we have about the brain is framed by a set of philosophical conceptions of humans and their relationship with the rest of the universe.[16]

Mental aspects of the brain are examined by other disciplines, such as psychology and psychiatry. Psychology studies the behavior of humans and their way of perceiving, thinking, reasoning, and so on. Psychiatry studies psychic or mental phenomena and behavioral deviations of individuals concerning the behavior of the average individual. On the other hand, philosophy plays a crucial role, as it critically examines the foundations of fundamental beliefs and analyzes the basic concepts used in the expression of such beliefs.[17] The mind is the brain in action.

From the Philosophical Point of View

Since humans acquired the capacity to reason, they have been eager to know and locate themselves in the universe and have asked questions about its origin, nature, and purpose. This has allowed us to form concepts of ourselves and the world around us, concepts that, in turn, have determined our attitude toward life. We could say that from the philosophical point of view, the interest in knowing the mind is ancient and that the first tool used to infer the characteristics of its functioning was introspection.

Perception

The way we perceive our surroundings is vital. Having feelings is an innate ability; we are born with it. On the other hand, perception is an individual capacity and of a personal nature, since it is the result of learning. As such, it depends on unique experiences, environment, and our own characteristics.

---

[16] http://bibliotecadigital.ilce.edu.mx/sites/ciencia/volumen2/ciencia3/088/html/sec_9.html.

[17] Ibid.

There are no natural connections between the auditory identification of a sound produced by an object and its visual identification. All these associations of ideas must be established through experience, and they form an essential part of the learning that takes place in young children. Hence, the importance of children growing up in enriched environments, since early expertise is of great significance in perceptual, intellectual, and emotional development.

Meditation

In meditation, I found profound insight; it is a technique that implicates understanding the nature of mind and self, as well as applying the insights gained in our relationships with others. From a spiritual point of view, the mind also represents the development of ego, as well as aspects of human intelligence, perception, and cognition. Actually, emotions can be recognized as an energy that affects, for good or for bad, the complex states of mind that we create.

Many techniques are used for meditation: Buddhist meditation, Transcendental Meditation, mindfulness, Vipassana Meditation, mantras, ThetaHealing, among others. Basically, through meditation we may answer questions we have asked for centuries: Who am I? What am I? Why am I? Preformulated answers seem to leave us unsatisfied. Meditation is an ancient technique, yet it is amazingly applicable and appropriate to working within our contemporary situations. It resonates with many of the discoveries of psychologists and neuroscientists.

Surprisingly, it is through meditation that some insights might arise when examining our own experiences, to such a level that we may be aware of what we think of as the self or our egos. Meditation is a discipline that requires learning from a non-ego point of view. Therefore, is based on opening your heart and discovering this natural sense of discipline. It is the discipline of educating yourself without ego, and it is also known as training your mind. You might think, "Sounds great—but how am I supposed to do that?" No worries. I'll get there.

ThetaHealing

Although meditation came into my life almost twenty years ago, I failed to have the necessary discipline to make meditation part of my daily routine. I became a mother, and suddenly I was absorbed with my children, plus many other things. I didn't commit myself to practicing meditation religiously, just to give myself some time to quiet my mind, even though I needed to silence it because I had a hamster spinning the wheel of my mind, twenty-four/seven.

Nevertheless, I found ThetaHealing when it was meant to be. I learned about this meditation technique a few months before I knew about my diagnosis. I always had considered the intellect of more importance than the spiritual, and I frankly had many doubts about what I heard of ThetaHealing.

I already knew that something was wrong with my health when fate led me to meet Lory A., who explained the ThetaHealing technique to me. I thought it was a dubious technique. It did not resonate with me at that time, but a couple of months later, pushed by curiosity (which I now know was my instinct), I asked her for a session.

During the session, things came out about my life that Lory could not have known. She worked on the limiting beliefs that had affected me since my childhood, beliefs that I unconsciously adopted throughout my life. Some of them, over time, became wounds. Because I couldn't see those wounds, I wasn't conscious of them, but they hurt when I encountered specific circumstances. It was painful, but it was a pain that was difficult to recognize, to feel, or to put into words, even as it manifested itself.

At the end of the session, I felt disoriented, like I'd just gotten off a roller coaster, and the effects of the shake remained for a time. I lost my cardinal points for a while, but I felt light and clear, emotionally. After a week, I discovered myself, assuming my day-to-day difference. For example, there was a family situation in which I suddenly realized that my way of dealing with it was entirely different from it used to be. I realized there was a *before* my first session of ThetaHealing and an *after*.

A few days later, I started with the exams to figure out what was happening with my health. This process lasted about a month, and when I learned of the cancer diagnosis, I started having panic attacks. At that time, Lory told me that she was going to teach the ThetaHealing Basic DNA course. I decided to take it because I knew there had already been changes in me, and I had to do something drastic in the face of such a devastating diagnosis. Once again, my intuition came to the rescue, so I started the journey of this technique at the same time as the first chemotherapy.

In this first course, I understood the processes from its beginnings. I also learned the story of its founder, Vianna Stibal, who, in August 1995, was diagnosed with bone cancer. Upon receiving the news that doctors would have to amputate her leg, she decided to follow her intuitive skills to heal herself—and she achieved it! This seemed intellectually unlikely but intuitively attractive, so despite the physical discomfort caused by chemo, I drew strength (I do not know from where) to continue my studies in ThetaHealing.

When I took the Advanced DNA course, I had just received the second chemotherapy. My husband and children took me to the course and almost carried me to the classroom. It was teamwork—someone brought my meal, someone else carried my purse. My physical strength was minimal, but my intuitive strength was what pushed me.

Discovering that inner strength is one of the things I most appreciate from ThetaHealing. During this advanced course, I was literally sleeping in my chair. From time to time, to everyone's surprise—and to mine—I would wake up to ask questions about what was being discussed. On the last day of the course, I felt an inexplicable vitality. In the final group photos, I jumped out, smiling, laughing—*alive* again.

Let me explain ThetaHealing; it is a meditation technique that seeks the connection of mind, body, and spirit. Throughout the years, through hypnosis, many people have been helped to come to a *theta* state with excellent results of improvement in their health. In ThetaHealing, it is posited that when a person can make a connection with the Creator of all that is (the divine within) through the state of theta, the healing or solution of that which is in us is attained.

The brain has five different wave frequencies—alpha, beta, gamma, delta, and theta. These are in constant motion in such a way that the brain continually produces all these frequencies, which regulate everything we do and say (from an electrical point of view).

The state of theta is one of deep relaxation and is the one that activates when we are in a hypnotic state. The wave frequency is reduced from four to seven cycles per second. It is said that the frequency of theta is that of the subconscious state. It governs the middle layer between the conscious and the unconscious mind and keeps memories and sensations. It also regulates attitudes, beliefs, and behaviors. It is believed that this state allows us to act on the level of the conscious mind. It is a mighty state.

Remember, we all are intuitive. And it is through the technique of ThetaHealing that intuition is developed much more. It's as if we suddenly open the door wide to our own universe, our spiritual world, which connects us directly with the divine, the Creator of all that is. No matter what your religion or religious beliefs are, this meditation seeks to connect with the spiritual body that all human beings have innately. Some people may not have explored this; others will have. What is sought in ThetaHealing, however, is that connection and superconsciousness of the existence of a spiritual body. It does not attempt to impose terms or beliefs of any religious type.

You may be wondering how ThetaHealing works. In a theta state, what we say and think is magnified, as we are in a state of superconsciousness. What happens there is imprinted at a cellular level and becomes a belief. That is why we must be careful with what we think, as it will have it consequences, for good or evil. The words we say also have an incredible effect in our daily lives.

Psychologists, pedagogues, philosophers, and studies on the subject of the psyche suggest that the most vulnerable age of a human being is between two and six years. This is because at that stage, the wave frequency that prevails most of the time is theta. It is a crucial stage because we are in a state of superconsciousness, where everything that happens is marked forever. All learning is recorded, every emotional event is recorded, every achievement, every trauma—everything is registered.

The more you develop your intuitive skills with ThetaHealing, the more your words, thoughts, and belief systems will have the power to make changes in your life—for better or for worse. You should understand that you are co-creator of your life, your destiny, and your reality, together with the Creator of all that is.

How can your thoughts affect your reality to such a level? The answer seems both exciting and complex, and for this, I will delve into quantum physics.

Quantum Physics

Max Planck is considered the father of quantum physics. In 1944 he caused controversy by saying that the DNA of life and the birth of stars arise in a place called *Divine Matrix*. It is in this matrix where all things originate; it is a place of pure energy, where energy simply *is*. Recent studies indicate that this matrix is real. For many scientists, this theory is the bridge between imagination and reality. Where our beliefs reflect into reality: they function as mirrors.

A lot of research and literature on the theory of quantum physics is based on a new vision of being, where everything existing is interpreted as energy in different forms of manifestation. According to quantum physics, when an organism loses its capacity to maintain its corresponding function harmoniously, the disease appears; this malfunction can be expressed in any tissue or organ. Therefore this reason is said that each person develops and manifest a condition or symptom.

When our imagination and our reality agree, it is said that miracles occur—miracles, such as the range of possibilities to travel in this life, or the possibility of a spontaneous healing of a disease, or the connection with everything that surrounds us; that is, knowing and recognizing ourselves as part of the whole.

From the traditional scientific perspective, we are passive observers of our reality; we are alien to it. However, from the perspective of quantum physics, we are co-creators of our reality. Thoughts have an energy that emanates a frequency which attracts the intention of that thought. That is why being aware of our recurring thoughts is a significant step forward in knowing what changes should be made to our highest best.

It's crucial to know how to connect with the divine matrix to improve our lives and, hence, those around us. Do you realize the importance of this? We do not recognize the potential we have as human beings. We are perfect machines; we are a microcosm in close relationship with the macro-cosmos.

For some reason, we are made to believe that we are isolated beings, that we are separated from each other and our world. This belief, to a certain extent, has made us feel like victims who aren't responsible for their suffering. However, have you noticed how a community responds to a natural catastrophe? Suddenly, the collective unconscious of the community is connected through compassion and empathy for others. Human beings connect with the collective belief that we are all one. Human beings respond from their essence to common situations.

But what happens once everything returns to normal? We are again isolated individuals.

Maybe this concept of the divine matrix will break the paradigm of your belief system. There is always the option to get out of your comfort zone and put this scientific concept to the test. The literature on this subject is extensive and based on scientific evidence.

Gregg Braden, in his book *The Divine Matrix*, writes the following:

> "It seems that we are the very energy that is creating the cosmos, as well as the beings that have the experience of being creating. This is because we are consciousness, and consciousness seems to be the substance from which the universe is made"[18].

The experiments of quantum physics unquestionably show that consciousness has a direct effect on the most basic particles of creation, and we, as human beings, are the source of consciousness.

I hope that this concept of divine matrix is causing questions and breaking paradigms. If so, it is a good start in realizing the importance of your thoughts (consciousness) and their effect on your reality. I hope you realize you are co-creator of your reality (like it or not), although you might utterly reject this whole idea, and that is valid as well.

In the end, life is based on decisions, and we have the free will to choose what to believe and what to think. Each of us is free to decide the appropriate changes to have better health, improve interpersonal and/or loving relationships, improve professional path, generate more income, or just remain the observer of what happens around us, oblivious to the facts that keep us out of balance in different areas of our lives. Dear reader, what do you choose?

Taking Action

I've shown the theoretical and scientific approach to the power of thoughts, but how do you adjust this information to your current situation? It is not necessary to have a health crisis (such as cancer, depression, anxiety, etc) to become aware of the effects of your

---

[18] Braden, Gregg. *La Matriz Divina: Un puente entre el tiempo, el espacio, las creencias y los milagros.* Editorial Sirio, S.A., 2009.

thoughts on your body and reality. Let's say this information is preventive medicine.

Currently, professionals in the scientific and philosophical areas have explained—very clearly and with evidence—the effect of thoughts on our reality, including Dr. Joe Dispenza, Lynne McTaggart, Bruce Lipton, PhD, and Gregg Braden, to name a few. Each one has had the passion and intelligence to convey the concept that Max Planck proposed seven decades ago, despite the criticism of Albert Einstein himself, who had a deep understanding of physics but kept it removed from the spiritual realm.

Vianna Stibal, developer of ThetaHealing, applies this concept of reprogramming new beliefs and discarding limiting beliefs.

In his book, *You Are the Placebo*, Dr. Joe Dispenza shares several documented cases of people who were able to reverse cancer, depression, and other diseases through believing in the placebo. He states that beliefs can be so strong that even drug companies use double or triple randomized studies to exclude the power of the mind over the body when it comes to evaluating new medicines. Dr. Dispenza explains the way in which our brains can produce the necessary substances to positively affect our physiology in such a way that our lives can be transformed.

"Be the alchemist," Dr. Dispenza states. Our personal, family, and social history show us a reality that is far from being the real one. Mind and matter are related to what reality can modify. For there to be a real change, we must understand how to generate it from the way we set our intentions to obtain results according to what we want.

Bruce Lipton, PhD, proposes a new field of traditional biology known as "the New Biology." In his professional experience as a teacher in medicine and as a scientific researcher, he has researched in depth the mechanisms in which cells receive and process information. In these investigations, he has discovered that genes and DNA do not control our biology, as has been maintained in the last centuries. Far from the theory that genetics defines us, he argues that DNA is controlled by signals outside cells, such as positive or negative thoughts as energetic messages emitted by the individual.

Lipton's experiments and studies summarize the best of cell biology and quantum physics, which proposes and demonstrates that our bodies can change if we reshape our thinking.

Lynne McTaggart, who has a background as a journalist and researcher, was immersed in this exciting world of quantum physics and healing. As a researcher, she was curious to understand the effects of quantum physics as a result of miraculous healings. She has dedicated the past years of her professional life (and I would dare say also her personal life) to travel the world, carrying out group-healing experiments. To her surprise, she not only saw the positive effect on people who receive prayer or meditation, but she saw more progress in people who meditate or pray for others. This fact captivated her and motivated her to write her book, *The Power of Eight*.

McTaggart has been recognized as one of the pillars of the new science of consciousness and as a spiritual person of an enormous influence in the world.

I find her proposal fascinating—that when a group of people concentrates an intention on a target, a powerful, collective dynamic emerges, which can heal (even over long distances) health problems and violence, to name just two. She scientifically demonstrates the miraculous effect of healing on the people who emit the prayer and those who receive it.

The Choice Is Yours

The prominent people just mentioned have taken action investigating and putting into practice a theory that emerged in the 1940s, a time in which human beings were not yet prepared to elaborate on this scientific concept. I have always thought that the era of homo sapiens must end to make space for the era of *homo spiritus* (a term I coined) or *homo divinus*. In my view, reason must give way to the spirit. I do not believe, however, that reason should disappear; on the contrary, it must work hand in hand with the spirit to complement the very objective of being.

The spiritual factor is intrinsic to being, but in general, it has been made a side factor. In some cases, it has been replaced by religion. Let's be honest—throughout history, there have been atrocities committed in the name of God that have come against the nature of the individual's spirit. I respect all religions, although I am not questioning them. When religion is not well understood, some religious institutions may use religion as a way to control and achieve power over others. Once in a while, they might use fear to control. The spirit manifests itself in different ways—in the arts (painting, music, dance, etc.), in compassion, in empathy to others. Once in a while, however, reason runs over the spirit. Sometimes, when in a survival mode, the balance of being is lost—a balance between mind and spirit. How do you know which one to turn to?

The choice is yours. Do you want to experience the effects of quantum physics? Are you willing to make way for your era of homo spiritus? Do you think that life has put you between a rock and a hard place? Or have you led yourself to such a situation in your life that you have to decide which path to take? Should it be the road on the left or the one on the right? What does reason tell you? What does your spirit tell you? Do you want to make changes in your life but don't know which ones?

For years, I was guided by reason. Eventually, I used more intuition (spirit) to make some decisions. As I grew up, I started to silence my inner voice. But then the diagnosis of cancer came, and this was a watershed moment in my life. Somehow, I was forced to give way to my own era of homo spiritus. I had nothing to lose, as the imminent presence of death was in front of me, prowling. It was then that I started ThetaHealing sessions with daily meditations, in which I focused my attention and intention on the perfect functioning of my cells, reaffirming that my body (like all human beings) has the wisdom and capacity for self-healing.

Talk to Your Cells

One day, I received a message on my cell phone from a friend who told me to talk to my cells. She gave me an image with an explanation. It seemed empirical to me, so I did not pay attention to it. The next day, however, I saw the message again and decided to trust that what I was about to do would be worthwhile. And so I talked to my cells daily for a few days, until it became a habit, and I no longer needed to follow her instructions.

I was already doing certification in ThetaHealing, and I was making sense of this ritual. After a while, I took a course called Intuitive Anatomy, in which I learned the hidden beliefs in each system of the body. I understood much more of the miraculous biological machinery we have and its function. Above all, I had the ability to visualize my meditations in action. While talking to my cells and commanding them to do their optimal work to achieve my healing and balance in health, I witnessed my biology working as I spoke.

During one of my visits to the clinic in Reno, my doctor explained how the chemical principle of chemotherapy would interact with my biology. He emphasized that he wanted me to imagine everything he had explained to me while I received the medication. That idea seemed excellent to me—visualize my cells doing their innate function. Wonderful! I was absolutely into it.

In 2004, I watched the movie *What the Bleep Do We Know!?* I found it extraordinary. It resonated with me. One of the scenes I remember most is when the protagonist was waiting at the subway station after she saw an exhibition of Masaru Emoto's "The Message from Water". This film was one of the first approaches I'd seen to quantum physics. Emoto was a Japanese researcher who experimented, by observing through the microscope, with how water molecules react when they receive the vibration of classical music, love words, or just the opposite. He demonstrated that molecules in a positive and loving environment formed perfect mandalas (perfect, sacred geometric figures). Water molecules in a negative and violent environment, however, showed amorphous and obscure figures.

If we consider that 75 percent of the body is water (as is the planet), what effect does a harmonious environment have on our own ecosystems? And what effect does an adverse environment have? (The same question would apply to our planet.)

From this theory, many people like to write an intention on their glasses or bottles of water for those molecules.

I did the same in my intravenous treatments. Of course, I had no way of checking the effect on my cells, but the words I wrote had a positive effect on my psyche and my spirit. Generally, I wrote the following:

- I am perfect health
- love
- strength
- determination
- inner peace
- light
- I trust my potential

The nurses already knew that it was my habit to do this, so they had everything ready for me to write on the intravenous bags. Soon, other patients started doing the same.

Now, my cells and I are in close communication. We have a healthy relationship, and we work as a team for our best. If I feel tired or have discomfort, I give myself time to meditate (in addition to my daily meditation) and talk with them in such a way that I reinforce their intrinsic function of returning to the natural balance of my health. Given all the information I've learned in this regard and the scientifically proven cases that demonstrate changes in beliefs and therefore in biology, I rely on this method widely. This is not the only method, however, I have used to heal. Remember I mentioned the importance of food, among other elements that complement the whole process of healing.

Manifesto

The word *manifesto* has its etymological origin in the Latin *manifestum*, which means clear or evident. A manifesto is intended to be a statement of a personal opinion, motives, or intentions. It serves as a way of decreeing what is essential. For some people, writing a manifesto is an act of rebellion; for others, it's a way of setting a precedent for something that is intended to be done. It is a commitment to oneself. But a manifesto can be a source of inspiration to meet the goals set by each person.

As individuals, we set particular goals, and these can change from time to time. It depends on what we want to achieve.

Sometimes after meditation, I write in my journal, do art journaling, or create a manifesto, which I read daily, so I have it present throughout the day as a reminder to keep my intention pointing to one direction. Other times, I need to change my manifesto because during the meditation, a new idea or a new goal arose. All my reflections are aimed at achieving balance in perfect health, but if that day I have a blood test or an important work meeting, or if I know I'll have to attend to a complicated client case, I go to the manifesto tool.

This exercise has been beneficial for me. Many times, I write it and put it in my workplace within my sight. Or if I feel that my mind is wandering or that some thought or negative emotion wants to take over me, I go to my manifesto, and—almost like magic—I return to the course of that day and recover my power.

The manifesto is useful especially if you are going through a complicated moment in your life, in which concentrating or finding direction is tough. It can act as a kind of beacon that tells you the safest way to get to what you want. As simple as it may seem, establishing—manifesting—your goals in writing generates a mental clarity and inner peace, as you unconsciously develop affirmations or reaffirm what you think is necessary at a specific stage in your life.

Your manifesto could be written, or it could be a drawing. (I'll explain more about creating an artistic manifesto in chapter 7.)

Think about what to write in your manifesto, and start from there. You'll need to choose a theme. In my case, it was decreeing my total healing, generating positive thoughts, and avoiding toxic people and foods. The word *no* is forbidden in the manifesto. Once the topics are established, you can write them in the form of motivation, intention, or positive belief. Below is an example of a manifesto, based on my goal of perfect health:

I trust in the natural power of my self-healing body.

I avoid toxic environments.

Despite the daily tests, I have the strength and the intelligence to get ahead.

My mind generates positive thoughts for my highest best.

I free myself from fear.

I live my life with fullness.

Exercise

Write down your manifesto. Write a letter to your cells.

Chapter 6

THE SPIRITUALLY
INFINITE JOURNEY

*Intuition is a natural sense that we have, but it is a "survival
instinct." Higher guidance is an earned spiritual relationship—
one that is developed between your soul and the Divine.*
—Caroline Myss

What Is Spirituality?

So far, I have addressed tangible matters; they have form and/or are
verifiable. Spirituality, however, is sometimes ephemeral, something
to which some people turn only when necessary. It could be ethereal
too because it complements the being that inhabits in our interior.
Some people, however, don't have an awareness of it, or they have
chosen, based on their own histories, to use their intellect more; that
is, there's a tendency to analyze everything that happens.

Spirituality produces an inner transformation. Those who work
adequately have a profound sense of spirituality. They know that
their qualities and the world in which they live cannot be explained
if they don't transcend their limited realities. Spirituality, faith, and
the unknown are inseparable in every aspect of life.

The spirit is an essential part of the purpose of life. It is what
drives us to keep going, even in the most challenging moments. The
spirit is the recondite part of our beings, the ultimate motivation, the
ideal, the passion, the mystique for which we live and fight and with

which we infect others. And it manifests in one way or another. It is always there, although we do not want to give it credit.

Throughout my healing process, I have had several moments of vulnerability—fear and uncertainty. But I also have had a strength (like an engine) that brought me forward in every moment when I needed it—it's that force that suddenly arises from nothing and nowhere. I could say almost exactly in what part of my body I feel it and even tell how it is.

The image that comes to my mind in those moments of darkness is a weak flame that seems to be extinguished at the slightest provocation. But when I give myself a moment (which may be days) of silence, or I withdraw from the circumstances of others and the outside world, I focus on that flame and start to fan it, as one who fans a bonfire on its last breath. And it is precisely in that silence that I let myself surrender and trust in the darkness that will bring me to the light. When we truly surrender, we reach a point where we are nothing, nobody. There is no time. There is no place, and we are simply consciousness.

That's when I see and feel that force of fire that takes a second breath and drives away darkness. Light opens the way for peace, confidence, and clarity to make the right decisions in choosing which path to take in each deviation that is presented. This happens because it is a state of being more focused on the spirit than on the ego.

It's not easy, but in the most challenging moments, I hear a voice that says, "Your spirit is strong," and then I repeat it to myself as an affirmation: *I am a strong spirit!*

Humans are fundamentally spiritual beings. The more consciously individuals live and act, the more they cultivate their values, ideals, mystique, options, and depth, and the more sense and understanding they have of being. For those who have more spirituality, their inner sources will be more profound and stronger. Spirituality is not exclusive to special people; it is present in all of us.

Spirituality implies an awareness of everything there is and an openness to reality. It is the strength that allows us to transcend reality and go beyond ourselves.

It is imperative to distinguish the spiritual from the religious dimension; it is not about separating but identifying. Spirituality is more extensive and is expressed in all people, even those who do not have a specific religious creed. Religion is the result of a relationship that has to do with the meaning of our lives and values.

Spirituality has to do with experience, not with doctrine, nor with dogmas, nor with rites, nor with celebrations. These are institutional paths that help, sooner or later because they were born of our spirituality.

Our challenge consists of discovering how to move from reason, where the doctrine of God is, to the heart, where the living reality of God (the divine) is found.

One of the significant contributions of spiritual understanding is that it reconciles the sense of self to something we might not imagine exists inside us. Spirituality states that despite the fact that we think we're limited and little, that is false. We are greater and more influential than we ever could guess. A great and divine light exists within us, and this same light is also already in our knowledge. We regularly think that we are limited to our physical bodies and circumstances, including our gender, race, family, work, and status in life, but spirituality emerges every day to make us aware that there is much more than the materialistic approach. In other words, it is beyond whatever we perceive through our five senses.

Moreover, the spiritual way is to see beyond external appearances. It's a path that takes you to the state of connecting with the universe and, at the same time, being part of all—oneness; being nothing and at the same time everything. It's knowing how to interact with the circumstances from an intuitive perception. Those who are more aligned with a spiritual approach may transform and expand their world to live in harmony and inner peace and to be aware of the well-being of themselves and others. Furthermore, they understand how to live in balance and in the present moment.

Trust Your Truth

I mentioned that I've heard a voice saying, "Your spirit is strong." We regularly listen to voices in our heads. These voices can be a messy chattering, but there is only one that is our truth.

Once we manage to recognize the voice of our truth, we see that the one who is speaking is our intuition—our essence, the light that guides us and motivates us to move forward. Throughout our lifetimes, we build a belief system influenced by our environment (family, school, work, society, marketing, socioeconomic level, etc.), and we might disagree with what surrounds us and with what we think we are.

Have you ever felt that you don't belong to a place? Despite any effort you make, there is just something that prevents you from relating to a particular type of people? Of course, we often make an effort to coincide ideologically and to feel the sense of belonging; we use masks according to the situation and place. However, those masks are only the facade we use to be accepted and not judged. But there is something inside that does not deceive us and that makes us see that we are not who the mask portrays.

This voice is the voice of spirituality; it is what we intimately recognize as a guide in life. And if we are in tune with that voice—that is, with our divinity—then we can cocreate a reality according to our essence, to our truth.

It's easy, isn't it? Yes, it is! There is so much disturbance outside, however, that it does not allow us to focus on our silence. Many people are terrified to discover what is internal, or they just are not aware that there is a universe within each of us. They think it's better to buy the idea that we are what we have—cars, clothes, etc.—and we follow the social game, even though it may be solitary and empty.

But if we are able to hear our truth and be congruent with it, we can take our lives into healthy spirits, where we achieve that growth and transcend both individually and collectively. In this world, by the way, that is what is most needed—conscious and congruent inhabitants.

One of the most important things to trust in our truth is that we can make decisions, however hard they may be, with the conviction that it is the best for us. Whether the decisions are related to health, money, or work, our truth will set us free.

Faith without Actions Means Nothing

Faith without actions means nothing. This phrase came to mind one day after a meditation. I reflected on the meaning of it for hours. I really appreciated the guidance of Reverend F. Mann a close friend of mine, who helped me to reflect about this. Faith is a belief that is not based on proof, but just because you don't see or know about things doesn't mean they don't exist. With regard to a disease that people assume is incurable or difficult to cure, faith plays a crucial role.

Throughout my healing process, I witnessed (and continue to witness) people who pass from their disease (each case has its own history). I have also seen, however, miraculous cases of healing: colon cancer with liver metastasis, MS, people who managed to walk after receiving a medical diagnosis that they would never walk again, my own miraculous healing process from stage IV lung cancer—if you go by the book, I should have been dead a couple of years ago—and endlessly complicated cases. What is it that motivates people to move forward? Faith!

We are co-creators with God (the divine spirit), so anything can be done for us that he can do through us. There is always the possibility of being healed, or wealthy, or whatever you're looking forward to achieving, but we must have faith and, at the same time, take charge of our healing, if that is the case, in partnership with doctors or coworkers or family, depending on what we're hoping for. To achieve this, we must be centered and grounded and be able to listen to the inner voice—intuition. In other words, we should tune in with our spirits. It is not all our work, but it is not all His work.

Tuning into Faith

How do we tune into our faith? In my humble opinion, we need to understand the meaning of *I am*. For instance, to be able to tune an instrument, we will need a tuning fork. When hit, it emits a sound, a wave frequency. The instrument is tuned according to the sound emitted by the tuning fork. As human beings, we tune in with the wave frequency that our own "tuning forks" emit. That is our self, the wave frequency that we broadcast externally, which is stimulated by our thoughts and their coherence with our emotions. We are able to generate harmony in our lives when we are in coherence. Then we can sense and affirm what we depend on—a low or high frequency.

If we become aware that the wave frequency that our tuning forks emit is low, it may be that the people around us also tune into our low frequency; if the frequency is high, they will tune in high. This makes us an influence in our community for good or evil.

It turns out that *I am* is a direct relationship with the divine (Spirit in motion) within us. Remember—it is our essence, our wisdom, our truth. And if we start from this premise—*I am essence. I am wisdom. I am my truth*—we will make affirmations and positive prayers. As a result, the frequency of our tuning forks will be higher, and this will attract positive things to our lives.

But how can we produce this frequency? Affirmations are thoughts. Once we realize these thoughts, we must focus and feel the emotions related to them in such a way that we will achieve coherence between thought and emotion. As a result, the experience of this moment will affect the frequency that our tuning forks will broadcast.

There are only two frequencies (energies): low (fear) and high (love). If we affirm every day, "*I am* love," this will be the foundation of our belief system, and therefore, we will be able to attract whatever we like. *I am* is the seed with which we are born, and the fruit we reap will depend on the care we take with it throughout our lives.

The Labyrinth: Symbol of the Soul

I've been intrigued by labyrinths for years. For some reason, I feel attracted to them. Maybe it's the shape, the intricate design, or their inherent power. Perhaps they are like a magnet to me. I feel drawn to a labyrinth and hypnotized when I see one, and I just can't resist walking through it.

The soul is expressed in images, rhythms, and metaphors, and the labyrinth, as an archetypal image, is a visible manifestation of all of them. It has been used as a route of pilgrimage and as a universal tool of meditation by various spiritual traditions. The most known labyrinth is the one in the Cathedral of Chartres, built around the year 1220, in France. It is a cosmological mandala and lunar-based calendar. Its foundation is in the sacred geometry, that old art that gives serenity and balance to the emotions and the mind, such as mandalas.

The circle is universally recognized as a symbol of totality and unity, the spiral of transformation and growth. For instance, the labyrinth in Chartres is a circuit of eleven laps and one that always leads toward the center, without treacherous roads or risk of being lost, and returns to the exit. The way inward facilitates cleansing and quieting of the mind. The central space is a place of meditation and contemplation to remain receptive to the blessings of silence. The path out leads to the integration of creativity and the loving power of the soul in the world. The labyrinth becomes a mirror that answers questions about who we are and where we are in our lives.

This sacred geometry as a labyrinth is a pure, tangible manifestation of the universal God mind (divine). The process of moving into and meditating in a labyrinth holds unlimited spiritual potential. It automatically moves us closer to the wiser aspects of our consciousness.

If we use the labyrinth as a metaphor in our spiritual paths and growth, we could say that in the search for our essence or truth, even in moments of considerable doubt, it is necessary to walk the intricate path toward the center of the labyrinth. Once there, we must give ourselves the time and space to meditate in silence and then resume the course toward the exit. Life is cyclical, and a labyrinth can accompany each cycle. It is essential to make the journey of each labyrinth that is present in our spiritual paths.

Questions accompany your way to the interior of your self, and the way to the exit will come with the answers to those questions. The answers to your questions are inside you, and that is where you should search—inside the labyrinth—and trust that the answers will come in their divine time.

Embrace Your Essence

After several months, my blood tests indicated I was cancer-free. I decided to declare myself in remission, even though my oncologist preferred to take things more slowly. After I was clean for a year, however, the doctor agreed I was in remission. To his surprise, my body always responded quickly and positively to treatment, apparently faster than most of his patients. On a routine visit, one of the doctors at the clinic went through the results of my most recent blood test. He said, "What the heck is with your cancer? I just don't get it! Your blood chemistry is of a person who has never had cancer."

A couple of weeks later, a routine lung x-ray showed that the nodules were still there. They had not disappeared, and that worried the doctors, who insisted I return to the clinic for extra treatment. My inner voice, however, convinced me that more treatment was not what I needed. What I had to solve was beyond the physical body. So I refused once again to follow the known; I decided on the unknown.

I believe that life puts us to the test all the time. Life continually changes our plans so that we open our eyes and our hearts and make sure that we are exposed to the unknown. At the same time, we attract these situations. It seems that life keeps kicking us out of our comfort zones. There are different tests—illnesses, divorce, death, and so on—and we must be creative in solving whatever belongs to each one.

Here is what cancer taught me from the spiritual perspective: I knew my inner strength. I discovered that I could trust in myself. I understood the importance of listening and connecting with my body, of feeling and following my intuition, and of defending my innate and acquired knowledge, as well as defending my body.

I lost the fear of the unknown. Now I feel and see the unknown with excitement because I know that it brings teaching. To follow my instinct is to know myself, guided by something beyond me. I tune in to my truth and defend it. I love me before anything and have stopped sacrificing for others—this isn't selfishness. To love and care for others, we must know how to love and take care of ourselves.

I feel an impulse (have a passion) to investigate. I've learned the importance of humility and giving the ego the place it deserves. I do not act or speak from the ego but from the heart, and I avoid judging.

My truth has weight and strength. I know how to listen to myself from compassion and unconditional love. I practice empathy.

I understand the value of my existence and that of others. I am moving from theory to practice; that is, learning is not only in the reading of a book. I must absorb and put into practice what I have learned. I don't stay in the role of the philosopher. I move forward and apply whatever I learned—hands-on, mind-on, and spirit-on. I have the great privilege of knowing myself more, as well as my abilities. I have overcome my limitations. I understand what it means to detoxify in every sense—food, environments and toxic people, negative emotions—by setting healthy, firm, and loving boundaries.

I became aware of the here and now (present). I gained awareness of the energy that I broadcast and attract. I live with more sensitivity and intensity. I have attained spiritual growth, and I give it its place. I accept it.

I learned to express and sustain what I think without imposing it on others. I found my purpose in life. I won the recognition of an achievement that was challenging to obtain. I saw the opportunity to inspire and motivate others in their struggles, and this gives me a chance to help as much as possible. I learned to have a good attitude in any situation. I understand that life is about decisions, and I decided not to victimize myself with the disease but to confront it with strength and intelligence. I learned to be in love with life, and this is the basis of everything. I have embraced my essence! I understand and feel the wholeness.

But above all, I managed to reach my human potential—a potential that we all have and that makes us magnificent.

Part III

THE HEALING POWER
OF ART JOURNALING

Chapter 7

ART JOURNALING AS AN INTUITIVE TOOL

The creation of something new is not a accomplished by the intellect, but by the play instinct acting from inner necessity. The creative mind plays with the objects it loves.
—Carl Jung

About Art Journaling

Art journaling is as simple as using a journal (drawing images rather than writing one's thoughts) and finding a safe place to create and express. It is a place with no rules or expectations, a place to be reflective. It even could be a therapeutic venue. You can use any medium and play with all kinds of supplies, from crayons and markers to acrylics or watercolors. You're the boss. You can set an intention for the process (or not), or you can let yourself be surprised by the result. The main idea, when dealing with a health issue (or not), is to let go of stress, fear, or frustration or to merely express faith, hope, trust, happiness, or any other positive emotion. Everything is allowed.

Anyone can do it! You might choose to browse for art-journaling ideas if you need inspiration. In the end, this is a personal way of expressing yourself.

If you continue to do art journaling on a daily basis, you may find that you repeat some patterns. Those patterns could be your unconscious artistic mark. You may also repeat words or express thoughts, even messages. It doesn't matter; the art journal is a unique insight into you. It is a kind of registered trademark.

You don't need to have an artistic background, skill, or expertise. Just go with the flow.

Intuitive Art Healing

Intuitive art healing came to my mind as a concept that encompasses art as a healing tool. It is not necessary to know any artistic technique or to have an artist's background or skills. Art and creativity, as an expression, is something intrinsic to the human being.

Art that is processed from intuition—from the need to express—goes beyond any theory. From the time cave paintings (around 30,000 years ago), people found a way to communicate without words, making images and symbols that arose from the soul, the heart, and the intellect.

Art, in all its expressions, is a way of contacting the most sacred part of the artist, of the human being. Throughout history, there have been talented people in different artistic branches—Mozart, Rudolf Nureyev, Leonardo da Vinci, Maria Callas, Picasso, Van Gogh, Frida Kahlo; the list is endless. All expressed their purest truths through their talents. Some may have had difficult lives, but in the arts, they found a way to cope and express themselves and maybe even to heal their souls.

The arts have been present in my life since I was a young child. My maternal grandparents were classical musicians. My grandfather was a guitarist, and my grandmother was a pianist. My grandmother and my mother always have been passionate about the arts. They would take me to concerts and exhibitions whenever possible. I was not very excited back then; it seemed very dull for a young girl. Once I was there, however, I enjoyed it. I appreciate having been exposed to the arts since I was a child.

In my adult life, I enjoy seeing the infinite creativity of human beings. I am amazed to see how each individual has a particular way of assimilating life and, in turn, expressing it. My husband and I strive to expose our children to the fantastic experience of the arts.

I followed the innate need to express myself as an individual in art, and that motivated me to make art therapy my profession. Among my other studies, such as clinical psychopedagogy, neuropsychology, ThetaHealing, neurofeedback, neuroscience, and biofeedback, I am passionate about understanding human beings as a whole. I truly believe it's my vocation to accompany and help others.

Art as therapy implies that both the spirit and the psyche unleash their expression unconsciously. My role as a therapist has been to guide and accompany my patients in the creative process so that later, they will give a deep sense to their symbols in such a way that they can release what needs to be released or accommodate what needs to be relocated in their systems. I have witnessed the healing of conflicts in many of my patients in so many ways, as well as in myself.

When Art Exceeds Consciousness

It's not not my intention to lecture on anthropology, sociology, or psychology, but I will approach these topics superficially and from the place that I occupy in my system, influenced by my personal and professional experience.

The language of art is intriguing; it's earning to read between lines. There are universal symbols, but there also are personal symbols. It requires study and practice to decipher the hidden messages of art. It's not only about critiquing a painting or a sculpture, or interpreting it, or giving meaning to the creative process; it's also about delving into the different layers and nuances of it.

Colors, textures, shapes, voids, and lines play an important role. They are the grammar elements that give meaning to the expression from a very deep and unconscious place. This could come from the back of the mind or the soul. Likewise, writing is an art—poetry or prose. Other examples of art are music, dance, film, or digital art. All these are expressions of the soul that sometimes pass through the filter of the psyche or suddenly pour on canvas or paper as a raw catharsis on some occasions. Art works as a channel when words are not enough.

Cave paintings are an example of how human beings found a way to express themselves, to cope, to tell a story, or to entertain themselves by creating. Scholars, including as Carl Gustav Jung, the famous psychologist and psychiatrist, have been intrigued by the innate impulse of humankind to draw circles from an early age. Jung himself drew for several years in the most crucial stage of his life. His internal images, drawn on a daily basis, gave birth to one of the most renowned books, *The Red Book*. For some, it is the most influential work in the history of psychology.

The first primitive figure that people tend to make is a concentric figure, such as the sun or a human figure made of a circle and lines—a stick figure. Later, elaborated mandalas (sacred circles) as well as labyrinths were seen in almost all cultures throughout history.

Am I Creative? Ten Ways to Ignite Your Creativity

You are creative! We all are; creativity is an innate act. We were born with the gift of creativity, and whatever we do in different areas of our lives—cooking, taking shortcuts, solving problems—we are being creative, unconsciously.

When it comes to an artistic act, however, most people get blocked and feel they aren't creative or original. As with everything in life, it's a matter of exercising your creative muscles.

With painting or writing, we might encounter the blank-sheet panic, but there are ways to confront that silent monster that seems to challenge by staring at us—and sometimes I feel he's making fun of me.

If you feel stuck instead of creative, consider the ten ways to ignite your creativity listed below. Make an appointment with your creativity on a daily basis—ten to fifteen minutes is enough. Pick one or more of the following ideas. Forget about expectations, and do not judge. There is no pretty or ugly, good or bad. Go with the flow.

1. Sit down to do breathing exercises. Inhale and exhale several times until you feel peaceful. That will take you out of your survival state; that is, you can let go of fear, anger, frustration, or any other negative emotion. When we are in positive emotion, we connect with our creativity.

2. Take a moment to close your eyes and listen to your favorite music. With your eyes closed, try to follow the beat while you doodle on a blank piece of paper, try not to open your eyes. You can use markers, colored pencils, or crayons. Use only one color. Keep it easy. You can leave it just as a doodle, or you can look for shapes and color them.

3. Grab your journal and write whatever comes to mind; keep writing. You will be surprised to see that, somehow, you have created a story.

4. Stare at clouds, and look for shapes.

5. Watch people walking along the street. Create their personal stories, but do not judge. Judging is not the goal of this exercise. If there's a couple or group of people, imagine what they are talking about.

6. If you're having a struggle, and you feel there is no outlet, imagine that there is an outlet. Write about it.

7. Grab some magazines, and look for images that call to you. Ask yourself what attracted you to those images. Glue them on a piece of paper, and draw, paint, write, or whatever you need to do with it.

8. If you like cooking, look for recipes and make your own versions.

9. If you're thinking about changing the decor of a room, look in magazines, go to stores, or browse on the internet.

10. Go for a walk; this improves creative thinking. If you live in a peaceful place or near nature, listen to that. If you live in a noisy place, listen to calm music while you walk.

Envision Health

I believe in the power of visualization. When visualizing, the brain does not know if what it sees is real or imaginary. Even imaginary fear can paralyze us or cause panic attacks, but what would happen if we put positive images in our minds? What if we created images or "movies" of situations in which we believe there's no exit, but we created one?

Let's get hands-on: whatever health situation (or any situation) you're dealing with, envision that part of the body (or situation) that needs to to be healed. Check the internet for images of the anatomic functioning of that part of your body. In my case, I focused on the lungs.

After finding the right image, I begin my meditation. I envision my lungs working in perfect harmony and for my highest best. While envisioning, I start feeling how it is to be 100 percent healed; that way, my mind and heart are working together toward the same goal. When meditating, I have supplies handy to start art journaling. I don't care about the technique or if it's pretty. I just focus on creating whatever I envision during my meditation.

Whatever I have created does not always make sense to my intellect, but it does to my soul. Once in a while, I revisit my creations, and sometimes I read a different story from the original. I discover details that I didn't see the first time or the previous times. I find this fascinating; it's like playing a mystery board game. Nevertheless, most important is that I picture myself achieving my goal—healing. If you can't picture your goal, chances are you won't meet your goal.

This activity can take as long as you want, and the way you envision yourself reaching your goal may vary during your healing process. Remember we're impermanent. Bottom line: if you don't witness yourself in your mind as already healed, you might not be healed.

I encourage you to have an art journal where you can paint, draw, doodle, or write whatever you need, every time you need to express emotions provoked by your healing process. This process is full of ups and downs. I believe it's not healthy to suppress these emotions. If you know that your health improved in a particular moment, that's exciting! Draw it. Write about it.

If you didn't receive good news from your doctor, that may be overwhelming, so get rid of that toxic emotion—express yourself! See art journaling as a healthy venue for expressing yourself through color, form, letters, magazine photos, personal pictures, etc. You will be amazed at how releasing this can be. Your art journal can be your best friend, your confidant, the shoulder you cry on.

I have no idea what my journey through cancer would have been without having the amazing tool of art journaling. The best part is that creation comes intuitively—no rules, no fears, no judgments; just surrendering and pouring thoughts and emotions onto the paper.

Sacred Space

I highly suggest you create a sacred space. Why? Because in this space you will have an opportunity to connect to your inner world. Remember that your body is your temple, so through art journaling, you will express your inner world. Make this creative moment a ritual, and find a place for you to honor this moment.

Here are some recommendations for creating a sacred space:

- Choose your favorite music (it could be a playlist). Calm music is ideal, such as classical, Gregorian chants, New Age, mantras. I recommend music without lyrics, as that could be a distraction.
- Use your favorite chair, spot, or cushion for meditation. If you don't have one, just choose one.
- Aromatherapy is great for relaxing. I'm a big fan of essential oils, and incense also is excellent for evoking a peaceful environment.
- Some people like to create an altar with elements that have sentimental or spiritual value, such as candles, rocks, photos. If you like that idea, follow your intuition. On my altar, for

instance, I have a collage that I created of my lungs, 100 percent healthy and clean, something that I have envisioned since I was first diagnosed.

If possible make this sacred space also your creative space, as you will be pouring your soul, thoughts, and emotions into your art journal. Before meditation, have your materials at hand so you don't lose your meditative state, and you can start creating as soon as you finish your meditation.

Chapter 8

A JOURNEY THROUGH YOUR MIRROR

What you seek is seeking you.
—Rumi

The Magic of Artmaking

I believe that artmaking is a spiritual path, as it's a way to connect with the divine within. It is an unconscious experience in which we pour out our issues (emotions, thoughts, stress, etc.) and in doing so, we create images. It is an opportunity to play with anything that might be bothering or intriguing us. It can also be an expression of joy and thankfulness. By artmaking, we may raise any question and may find meaning in any situation. It is also a place of honoring whatever we're dealing with.

Artmaking is a bridge between two worlds—the spiritual and the intellectual; the language of soul and psyche's language; consciousness and unconsciousness. Overall, it gives new understanding through the creative process, and in doing so, it solves internal conflicts and expresses awe and reverence to them.

The fact of creating art is linked to the concept of the quantum field, in which time does not exist; there is no past, and there is no future. There is merely the moment of artistic creation itself. It is like being suspended in the immense and vast space of a canvas, a blank page, a stage, or any area ready for the magic of expression to begin. It's the most exciting experience of surrendering to the unknown because although you may or may not know what you are doing, you don't know in what this artmaking will result.

Why Artmaking?

By artmaking, we may become resilient as well because we can reach a state where we practice flexibility by being open to any result of our art. If we create art on a regular basis, we will recognize the connection between soul and psyche in the very process of creating. Furthermore, over time, this transmutes into wisdom because our belief systems may change, and therefore we will be more tolerant with ourselves and with others.

Artmaking involves creative energy that is nothing more than the pure expression of our divinity and its relationship with the outside world. It occurs in such a way that the images we create lead us to know or understand each other better. For this, we can seek to create with a conscious or unconscious intention by being open to creating more than with the pure intention of releasing what is bothering us. I believe that what you seek is seeking you, so in any case, the result will be what it is meant to be. There are no accidents in the creative process.

Intentional or Unintentional

There are two ways to begin artmaking: intentional and unintentional. By intention, you state your request as an expected outlet. You may start your process by writing a purpose for the act of creating art. This is useful as a guideline and to keep present during the process, but it doesn't mean that is going to happen as expected. During the process the soul and mind could give an unexpected twist, and you have to be open for that to happen. In fact, this turn can occur so discreetly that you won't notice it until the end of the process.

It is interesting to have the opportunity to write a testimony of the whole process, from the moment the intention is written until the creation is finished. In this testimony, seek to bring to the surface of consciousness everything that needs to be seen, in such a way that at the end of this writing, you will have managed to integrate what has appeared in artwork.

You might think unintentional is a much easier way to start creating, but for me, it is sometimes overwhelming. Looking at a blank page can be paralyzing. Starting to write or paint without thinking, however, with an empty mind is a good start.

Igniting your creativity can be entertaining because you may discover a talent that was hidden for years. Generally, the surprises are pleasant. It is also a challenge to surrender fully and flow with what is emerging without analyzing, judging, or questioning, and leaving later a space for later in which a dialogue between the creator and the creation begins. You will be impressed with your own hidden language.

Which is the right decision—intentional or unintentional? Both are valid and worth an experiment. You can decide which one is the best for you; even better, you can play it by ear. Listen to your inner voice, and choose whichever is the best method, depending on your needs.

Pouring Out Your Soul and Psyche: Imagery

What is imagery? Jeanne Achterberg describes this in her book *Imagery in Healing*:

> Imagery is the thought process that invokes and uses the senses: vision, audition, smell, taste, the senses of movement, position, and touch. It is the communication mechanism between perception, emotion and bodily change. A major cause of both

health and sickness, the image is the world's oldest
and greatest healing resource[19].

I affirm that you may see imagery as if it's a placebo, as a form
of a suggestion for those who need or want to heal.

I've discussed the power of thoughts and their effect on our
physiology. Images also play a crucial role as profound causes of
physiological change. In general terms, the imagination can make
us sick or heal us; in some cases, it could have a miraculous and
unexpected effect. Imagination as a healing phenomenon is a
powerful concept because it impacts our four bodies: emotional,
physical, mental, and spiritual.

The images affect the sensory systems, although these may vary
in their responses to the stimulus. Some people who experience
intense imagery may have equally fierce reactions. These images
can trigger memories of the past. These images can be evoked by the
imagination or by the sense of vision in such a way that it can cause
people to connect with an emotion that has a direct effect on their
physiology, causing sweating or palpitations, for example.

I feel if we are willing to use imagery as healing, we should
have a clear image (as clear as possible) of what we wish to heal.
As mentioned, the act of artmaking with intention, in this case, is
crucial.

If we are going through a moment of imbalance in health, then
in the intention, we should seek to return to a balance in health.
Creating an image of a specific part of the body that we want to heal
should be created with ways to develop it in perfect health, in such a
way that this will be the image that our physiology will obey.

You can make several versions of it, and all of them will have the
common factor of healing. Each creation will be different, and each
may have various meanings, but the aim will always be the same.

Art therapy plays a significant role as a high influence in the
treatment of chronic diseases such as cancer. Hospitals across the

---

[19] Achterberg, Jeanne. *Imagery in Healing.* Shambala Publications, Inc. 1995

globe have opened their doors (and minds) to art therapists for emotional support to patients who deal with these health issues.

I had the great fortune to use this method in my personal process and in other people's process with cancer. The results were amazing because by releasing stress, fear, and anguish with the simple fact of creating, people also have addressed and sought healing in the images they produced. Remember this has an effect on the physiology as well as the spirit.

Grasping the Ground

Because the diagnosis in my body was lung cancer, my imagery was centered in my lungs. For many months, my awareness was on breathing, on observing and feeling my lungs breathing to their maximum extent. I had to learn to breathe consciously. I followed the natural breath of babies. Through yoga, I found the harmonization and coordination of my body and my breathing. It was the same on my walks, and even now, there are times when become aware of it while eating or doing other daily tasks. My respiratory system, although it still loses its rhythm, is in excellent condition, given my past health.

This situation motivated me to create a painting (imagery) of my lungs to find a way to represent their function and meaning in my life (other than the anatomical function and definition). I had this image in my mind—my lungs as the roots of a big, healthy, and abundant tree.

A root's function is to nurture, to hold, and to take over, and it's a fantastic network, almost the same as a human brain's network. I found this similarity between brain and lungs fascinating. During this process, I felt confident and fluent as the paintbrush caressed the white paper that, little by little, began to be colorful and powerful. I loved the way the colors combined and worked together. Somehow, a starry night began to appear for me. This sky was peaceful and bright, kind of an invitation to be connected to the vast universe.

While painting the ground, my goal was to express the importance of being grounded, aware of the here and now and the source of strength and safety in life. Lungs, which actually represented my roots, gave such meaning to this painting. Roots are a representation of our origins, our tribe, our traditions, and they encourage a sense of belonging. As soon as I added the image of my lungs to the painting, as if by magic, the sensation was fulfillment and hope. I saw myself like that tree—alive, energetic, healthy, balanced.

What this image summarized was the union between mind, body, and soul (environment, tree, roots). I needed to *grasp the ground* to reach the sky, to reach my truth, and to find my purpose in that particular time of my journey. To the extent that I was aware of it, my life took on another meaning. The impact of the image was powerful and definitive in bringing me out of that labyrinth in which I was lost. (Fig.1)

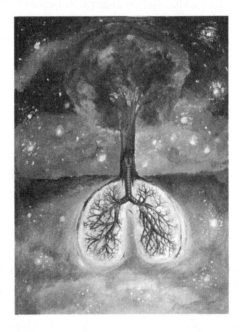

I created this drawing at a time when I needed some air, and I lacked space. I needed to feel I was in an open environment. When I lived in Barcelona, on some weekends I escaped to Montserrat. I would sit on a rock at the top of a mountain and spend hours contemplating the landscape. In those moments, I felt free and connected 100 percent with nature. In this drawing, I tried to recreate the scenes and the freedom I felt. In adding my lungs to the picture and creating them as big and transparent, in that moment I could feel my own lungs expanding and filling with pure air and freedom.

I drew falcons gliding in the emptiness of the sky. It gives me great peace to see their flight. I am intrigued by the flight engineering of birds as they fly.

The feeling of the final artwork, the sensation of connecting the interior environment with the exterior, was a reminder of that continuous interaction of both worlds. (Fig. 2)

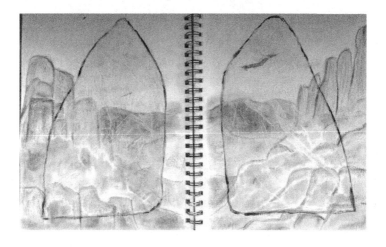

The need to make this painting came from the idea of visualizing big, green lungs (green is a symbol of health). The background has vibrant and intense colors that, to me, represent vitality, intensity, strength, and energy. This artwork honors my lungs. I included a small note to reinforce the image. (Fig. 3)

"I honor my lungs: I thank my lungs for every breath, for the oxygen that enters my body, because they know how to do their function divinely and the strength they have. My lungs are CLEAN and work

for my highest good. They are healthy, and they are love. They know how to receive and give love, health, and life. Thank you! Show it to me! It is done! It is done! It is done!

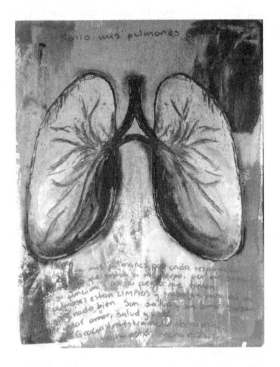

The following painting represents the power we all have to self-heal. It is not a self-portrait; it is the image of a healer. It could be me, you, or any other person, as we all have the innate potential to heal.

The process of this artwork was different layers of colors, shapes, and papers because that's how I think we are as human beings—layers of colors, layers of emotions, and layers of forms, and we play different roles in life. The black and white pattern paper represents the light/dark duality, yin and yang, our shadows and our light. There are also written words that represent the thoughts and stories from which we perceive life. The butterflies represent the transformation. Each challenge or stage of life brings with it learning and, therefore, a transformation. We leave the cocoon when we are ready to fly to the next unknown cycle. (Fig. 4)

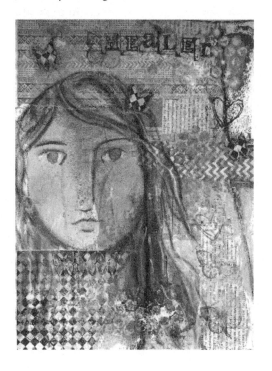

Lucky You!

Lucky you, if you think you cannot paint. You will have a spontaneous and unique way to create, despite never having done it before. It is likely that you have never had the opportunity to paint or write as a form of genuine expression. If you think you have no idea what to do, this is excellent news because you will have the opportunity to invent.

You can reproduce what you see in your mind, which can become a challenge and force you to abandon it, or you can invent from nothing and intuitively as it emerges. This is what I did in my painting of grasping the ground, letting myself be carried away by the brush. I did have an initial idea, but this was modified from moment to moment.

Not knowing how to paint gives freedom to create without the limits of the technique or what it "should be." Everything you show on the paper will be fresh, original, and unique.

I want you to know and understand the power of imagery but not feel overwhelmed by not having artistic talent. Remember that the critical points are to express yourself and the value that the final image has for you. The process is crucial because it is a path that you take to arrive at the solution to a problem.

Imagine that you are in a place that you need to leave for your sake, and you must go to another. There may be several ways; choosing the most accessible path sometimes does not give you the same satisfaction as selecting the most beautiful path, although it carries some difficulty. When you reach that desired place, the joy of the achievement will be such that it will have a substantial effect on your healing process.

Part IV

NO ONE KNOWS YOU BETTER THAN YOU

Chapter 9

CASES OF SUCCESS

Don't underestimate yourself. You have the ability to wake up.
You have the ability to be compassionate.
—Thich Nhat Hanh

In this chapter, I'll share success stories that I've had the good fortune to witness and to accompany the process. I am very grateful to the people who have allowed me to serve them and who have expressed their fears to such a degree that they have opened their hearts to me.

I recognize and honor their courage because I know that it is *not* easy to encounter the monsters that sometimes don't let go of us, without realizing, though, that we are the ones who have the power to let them go.

I also thank the people who allowed me to share their cases in this book. For me, all cases are successful; I saw myself in the difficult situation of choosing only some cases. Out of respect for them, I do not use their real names.

Even though I was told by a doctor that I was a "sad case", as mentioned earlier in this book, I was sure though, that I was a success story because in my soul, it was clear that I would get ahead of this condition. I believe we must know ourselves as doers, deserving and successful in any area of our lives. This process is not only to get out of a health problem. It applies to everything!

Alexa's Case

Alexa had surgery scheduled to remove fibroids from her uterus. She tried for a couple of years to treat them in an alternative way, but the fibroids still grew, so she and her obstetrician decided to remove them before they could hinder the functions of other organs and become complicated.

Given this circumstance, she knew it was the correct decision, but the idea of surgery caused her anxiety. It seems natural that the procedure would cause stress, anxiety, or fear. It is not fun to think of exposing yourself to a vulnerable situation.

Nonetheless, Alexa says that I helped her to address this anxiety. In reality, she helped herself by understanding her potential. She had anxiety before the surgery; she was terrified of any intervention— having her blood drawn, thinking of dying or having a terminal illness. All that faded after a ThetaHealing session.

I assisted Alexa in her preoperative process. In this, we focused on finding the fundamental belief of her anxiety, which emotionally and symbolically involved the uterus, and what could represent these myomas (tumors) at the emotional level.

Once all these beliefs became conscious, and they made sense to her, we began to program new beliefs that would work for her highest good, in such a way that her body would not resist the procedure and could let go of the myomas easily.

Remember that cells have emotional memory, so by guiding Alexa through meditation with the ThetaHealing technique, those memories were erased and healed. The information from the cells was replaced by beliefs that made her feel emotionally and physically ready. Her fear of death and diseases disappeared, as well as her fear of airplanes that also gave her a lot of anxiety.

At the end of the session, Alexa was ready for surgery. I suggested we give the fibroids permission to leave her body, and I encouraged her to *see* them leave without resistance. She visualized the liberation of everything that those fibroids represented at the emotional and physical levels. The command was to visualize how her fibroids were removed without any resistance. More critically, she visualized that her uterus recovered perfectly and without setbacks.

The doctor removed more fibroids than those shown on the ultrasound—one was the size of a grapefruit. This prolonged the procedure much more than expected, and her uterus needed to be reconstructed. The obstetrician warned her that she could have abundant and prolonged bleeding and that it would take a few months before her periods became regular.

However, Alexa did not have abundant or prolonged bleeding, which is normal for a surgery situation, similar to a cesarean section. She had her normal period twenty-eight days after the operation without problems or pain or heavy bleeding (much less than expected). She did suffer some anxiety attacks after the surgery, but in the same way, we were able to have another ThetaHealing session to release that energy and let her body recover and normalize naturally.

A week after Alexa's surgery, the doctor could not believe his eyes! The recovery that Alexa had achieved was terrific; he did not even consider performing an ultrasound because there was no inflammation or any symptom that justified it. It was above all medical expectations.

Having been freed from beliefs that generated stress and uncertainty before the operation and visualizing a successful surgery was the key for Alexa so that she could make a bitter pill easier to swallow—an enriching and liberating experience in every sense.

I am so pleased by the great job that Alexa did to help herself. It was an excellent opportunity for her to prepare for her surgery at the emotional, mental, and even energetic and spiritual levels. All doctors ask for preoperative studies to see if the body is in optimal condition for the procedure, but no one ever checks on whether the emotional and/or mental state of the patient is ready for it.

Don't you think it would be fascinating to research the results of addressing emotional and mental states before surgery versus not having any support?

Doris's Case

Doris attends a weekly women's group that I am in charge of. There, she expressed several times that she suffered from headaches almost every day. In some of the activities that I led, she realized that she was repeating her mother's patterns—she always complained of headaches. Over time, Doris expressed her fears at an unconscious level concerning her health, mainly related to her head.

I always strive to make the group aware of the importance of thoughts in our health. There is a close link between what we think and its somatization. Thus, this has become almost like a mantra that I repeat in most of the sessions.

Doris stopped attending the group for a while. Her presence was intermittent until a year and a half ago, when we received the news that she had a stroke. Of course, the news impacted all of us as a group, as we had been together for almost five years. I was certain that somehow she had attracted this to her life unconsciously.

This happened in January 2017; a few days passed before we had a clear report of her health status. My co-therapist and I contacted Doris's brother for permission to send Doris a letter, and we asked him to read it out loud to her every single day. It didn't matter that she was in an induced coma because we were sure that she could hear (those things that your heart knows). In the letter, I wrote to her in the form of guided meditation with instructions for her body to regenerate naturally and that she was strong and her nature was wise. She was soon going to replenish.

Her brother agreed, and he read the letter to her daily.

Doris woke up a few days later. As expected, she did not know or understand what had happened to her. Her speech was not clear, and her body was clumsy, but it was restored, little by little.

After she woke up, I wrote a new letter, changing the commands for the late stage of her recovery. For a while, we did not hear anything about her.

One day, she appeared in the weekly sessions, walking on her own feet. We all jumped to hug her and greet her. The progress in her rehabilitation was impressive. She was still struggling to express herself verbally, however, and her movements were slow. Once again, she stopped attending the sessions for a while because it required a lot of effort to do so.

After a while, she came back again, and this time, we could tell she was another person. She looked much better, but during the session, she expressed how difficult it had been for her emotionally to walk through this process. She said that she had asked God to take her with him because she was losing all hope as well as patience. She told us that she despaired because the right side of her body wasn't obeying her.

In that session, I guided the group in meditation, in which I specifically asked Doris to visualize and feel that the right side of her body moved with fluidity; that she was able to see, feel, and handle the perfect balance between the two sides of her body; and that she could work in harmony as a whole and without resistance. I suggested everyone do this exercise at home whenever they felt the need to reaffirm positive beliefs and every time they felt despair, anxiety, fear, or any negative emotion.

A week later, Doris sent me a video of her driving for the first time since the incident. There were not words enough to express my excitement. She also sent me an audio message, saying she already was feeling her right side and that every morning, after her prayers, she could visualize and feel her right side working in balance with the rest of her body. She told me that she had lost her fears and now was feeling positive that she would soon have her physical and verbal abilities back.

I admire Doris because, like all of us, she is overcoming a challenge, and I see her determined to love herself and to be surrounded by the love of her family toward the final stretch.

Elsa's Case

Elsa has been part of the weekly women's group for about four years. I only learned of her case last year when she decided to stop attending. We learned of her struggle on the very last day I ever saw her.

That day, she shared that she'd had bulimia for almost twenty years, but she had never told anyone about it, not even her family. She tried several times with different therapies to cure this addiction. We were surprised by her story because although she participated actively in the group, she never had mentioned it at all.

She shared her gratitude for me and my co-therapist, as there were a series of activities (related to art therapy and systemic therapy, basically), reflections, and meditations on which she worked so profoundly that she managed to eradicate the roots of bulimia. She became conscious about the belief system she'd previously had and during the twenty years she'd had bulimia. She managed to reprogram positive beliefs into her new belief system.

I consider the day she expressed herself openly as her graduation. Although I have not seen her since then, and despite not being able to accompany her consciously in her process—we did address several issues but not specifically bulimia—Elsa is a success story.

Theresa's Case

Theresa was diagnosed with depression; she was relatively new to therapy. She usually was quiet, but she recently shared that she has been taking antidepressant and anxiolytic tablets for seven years. The doctors told her that there is no cure and that she will be taking pills for the rest of her life. She is forty-two years old and refuses that idea.

She said that despite what her doctors said, she has heard a voice inside of her saying, "There are other options for managing depression and anxiety."

I don't advise anyone to stop doing what the doctors tell them to do. On the contrary, I think it is essential to listen to doctors because they have vital preparation. I would never recommend to anyone to stop taking what they were prescribed.

But I let my patients know that nobody knows our bodies better than ourselves, and it is very viable to work as a team with doctors. We should lose the fear of asking questions and evaluating whatever has been proposed to us as treatment. It should be something we want to do or that somehow resonates with us. It's a sensitive issue, however, and making decisions should not be taken lightly.

In Theresa's case, I recognized that she'd had an awakening of consciousness, and this is an excellent event in anyone's life. She now knows that she has an inner voice, and if she listens to it, it will be a great guide in her life for any decision in any field. Therefore, although this awakening has just begun, Theresa is already a success story.

I could share many more successful cases, but I hope these few examples will inspire you if you feel unmotivated or believe that it's dark at the end of the tunnel.

I hope you can see yourself reflected in each of these cases. None of these people is special; even my case is not special. We are people who have discovered, in a certain way, the potential that we have. All human beings have a vast potential, ready to be used for our highest good. It is never too late to sink into our interior in search of that divine treasure that we all possess.

Chapter 10

PLEDGING TO YOURSELF

There is a voice that doesn't use words. Listen.
—Rumi

Healthy Boundaries

The most difficult word to say is *no.* Why? In my opinion, it is because we are afraid of offending or hurting someone if we say that we don't want to do something that's asked of us. In general, we have been educated to please others. In childhood, we learned to obey. However, on occasion, some things are against our principles or our essence. I believe there is a fragile line between good manners and doing what we feel is against us.

How can we know when it's okay to accept and when should we say no? It seems to me that there can't be a generalized response to this. Each individual has his or her history and way of seeing life. Even in the same family and when family members have had the same education, the perception of life can be very different.

I think choosing to refuse is based on having healthy self-esteem, knowing how to respect yourself, and, in some cases, using common sense. If, at a particular moment, a person or a group of people make you feel uncomfortable or invade your space, it is essential to set a healthy and respectful limit to protect yourself.

I watched an interview with research professor Brené Brown, in which she talked about boundaries. She said, "The most compassionate people are also the most boundaried."

What an interesting concept, and how truthful it is! We must be compassionate to ourselves to set our boundaries. Plus, it is closely related to self-esteem. High self-esteem is required to know where and when we need to set compassionate, fair, and reasonable boundaries.

Boundaries are needed in the physical, emotional, energetic, and mental realms. They determine what we agree—or disagree—to allow.

- Physical: Is it related to your personal space (body)?
- Emotional: Understand how to separate your emotions and responsibility. This will make you aware when you're blaming or accepting blame or giving advice when no one asked for it.
- Mental: With regard to your thoughts, values, and opinions, do you respect others' beliefs or ideas? Do you feel the need to impose yours?
- Energetic: Be aware of your elecromagnetic field.

Be the Best Version of Yourself

Imagine that you are a rough diamond that was extracted from a distant mountain of difficult accessibility. You are merely a virgin and hard carbon rock.

You are a crystalline made of carbon, caused by extreme heat and pressure. Metaphorically speaking, perhaps you have been exposed to severe challenges in your life. The word *diamond* comes from the Greek *adamantium*, which means "invincible." You are a natural mineral, considered the most valuable gemstone and the hardest natural material. Do you realize what I mean by this?

You Are Your Best Advocate

If you want to survive any kind of crisis, you must defend yourself. This does not mean that you must be in a constant struggle or fight. It is not about living in a defensive mode. In my opinion, it means to be aware of the red lights in your heart, your mind, or your spirit. To ignore these signals is to deliver control of your life or your health to an alien entity. As I have said repeatedly, only *you* know what really happens in your body.

It seems a great responsibility to learn to know ourselves. In general, no one educates us for that. For instance, if we present symptoms, they can be quieted with medicine, but in many cases, we need to get to the bottom of the symptom to eradicate the root problem. If we do not know ourselves, if we do not listen or understand the language of our bodies, if we turn a deaf ear to our hearts, then time will take care of making us face that situation, sooner or later.

I think it's vital that we teach our children to listen to themselves. We should give them, when the occasion warrants it, the opportunity to choose a solution for their problems. In this way, they will have the chance to make contact with their truth. In the same way, if they tell us they're feeling pain or distress, we must give them that credit so as not to silence their souls.

I want to share my personal story about how I understood the importance of advocating for myself. I have four children who were all born in natural childbirth. For my the birth of my first child, my oldest son, I was afraid that it would hurt or that something would go wrong. In that first birth, I learned that my pain threshold was high. I understood the communication that existed between my son and me during the process of giving birth. It was a great discovery, although in reality, despite having given all the power to my obstetrician's knowledge, I was able to discover new sensations in my body. This first experience took me an hour from beginning to end.

The second delivery was very fast. My obstetrician had left the delivery room for a moment, and the doctor left in charge didn't know what to do when suddenly my hip "thundered." I heard a loud crack and felt a tug on my head. Almost immediately, I began to tremble, almost to convulse. At that moment, I got scared. I looked at the faces of the people who were in the room, who also didn't know what was happening. I realized that if I tensed my body, as a reflection of fear, the tremor increased. Somehow, I realized that I was opposing the nature of my body, which needed to be relaxed so that my baby could be born. Something inside me told me that this tremor had to do with the loss of control of my nervous system as it passed through the spine, so I saw it, to some extent, as a natural process. All I had to do was relax as much as I could and trust that the doctor would arrive at any moment. That's how it was, and a few minutes later, I gave birth to my second son. It took almost thirty minutes to deliver him.

My third birth took around twenty-two hours. I'd taken a hypno-birthing course to be prepared for this birth. Throughout the course, I became aware that my baby and I would work as a team. It was a much more conscious pregnancy, and I understood, in depth, that a woman's body is designed for pregnancy, childbirth, and breastfeeding. It was expected that the delivery would be easy and fast, as the previous two births were very fast. As soon as my obstetrician realized that my cervix was beginning to dilate, he immediately sent me to the hospital.

Even though the dilation increased, my baby did not go down as expected. I resisted being injected with oxytocin to stimulate labor; in previous births, I had agreed to it, and the deliveries were too fast. I devoted myself to listening to my body so I could know what to do. As I expected, my doctor and my husband began to worry because things seemed to be taking longer than usual. After a few hours, I agreed to be injected with an antispasmodic drug, even though I wasn't convinced. After a few minutes, I started to show symptoms of an allergic reaction, and, once again, something inside told me that I should relax as much as possible, despite a migraine that I'd developed because my blood pressure was very high. I knew I was in good hands; I'd always trusted my doctor and knew he would do his work. I would do mine as well. Suddenly, a doctor began to apply acupressure to my feet to relieve the migraine symptoms. Then my blood pressure went to average numbers. Once they stabilized me, the doctor and my husband considerde the option of a cesarean section, to which I categorically refused. I knew I could give birth naturally.

The doctor, however, took the baton and started to prepare everything for a C-section, as my life or the baby's life could be in danger. He wasn't willing to take a risk. I asked him to give me a few minutes to relax. What I actually did was close my eyes and connect with my baby. I told her that I was willing to have a natural birth but that I needed her to work with me. I told her I'd give her a few seconds to decide because they were too many hours of work already. While doing this, the doctors prepared everything for the C-section. They had already inserted the anesthesia in my spine, and they were about to tie my arms, but I refused to allow it. Then the doctor rechecked my cervix dilatation because I felt that my daughter had begun the birthing process.

Everyone told me that sensation was the effect of anesthesia, but I insisted on being rechecked. My doctor, to whom I will always be grateful for his patience, agreed to recheck. It was probably to please me, as he was sure it was not true. To his surprise, the baby was ready to born! Now the medical team had to hurry faster because the plans had changed in the very last minute; it would be a natural birth!

One of the assistants told me I should wait because they were not ready to receive my girl, but I said, "Ready or not, here we go. My daughter and I are already." I began pushing, and everything went perfectly.

Fifteen months later, I gave birth to my fourth baby. This time, I felt confident about the communication my body had with my baby. My cervix began to increase a few weeks before the due date. I attended my doctor's appoinments every week. I was able to feel that my hip stretched slowly at nights while I was at home. Sometimes when I went to the bathroom, my husband was afraid that I would give birth there!

This time, I decided that I would go to the hospital when I felt it was time to go. My cervix was approximately three centimeters increased for two weeks, and then one night, I felt more pressure on the hip, and cramps were frequent and rhythmic. The next morning, I went to see my obstetrician, who immediately sent me to the hospital. This time, everything was very easy; it took four hours from the doctor's visit until I had my fourth baby in my arms.

For me, these four births marked the beginning of my consciousness between my body and my mind, as well my rights as a patient. They let me discover that we all have a divine right by nature, and there is an innate need to advocate for ourselves, to protect ourselves, and to know how to take good care of ourselves. I learned that the medical staff and I were able to work as a team. My knowledge and theirs both are valid and crucial.

It's not necessary to go through extreme cases to achieve the awareness of advocacy. Examples can range from deciding what to eat for a tummyache, to knowing if we should accept an invitation to dinner (or dating), or even to know what decisions to make in case of cancer.

Pledging to Yourself

Throughout this book, I've discussed different situations in which I've had advocate for myself when I felt a treatment was not ideal for me, so I looked for options. Sometimes the options popped up to me, even without my looking for them.

Knowing how to advocate for yourself is imperative, as well as knowing how to avoid toxic relationships, environments, and food. Understanding to establish healthy boundaries, even to knowing how to respect the limits that other people place on us, is crucial in life. It is a skill that we all have, and we should be aware of it and practice it a lot, as if it were a muscle.

Why is it important to pledge to yourself? Because to the extent that we know each other, we know our limits, and we know how to set them healthily. Knowing how to advocate for ourselves, without fear or guilt and with compassion, allows us to live with more confidence and enjoyment. We can make this pledge, in which we commit individually by self-love to take care of ourselves in any area of our lives, but we *must* love ourselves enough to do this.

Regardless of healthy boundaries, it's essential to observe ourselves and learn to know each other to establish our own limits. In short, we must live our lives more consciously, listen to our inner voices, and remain firm but flexible before the experiences that life presents to us.

We probably don't make the correct decisions sometimes. If this is the case, we can turn the page and be grateful for learning from the experience. We can see this situation as expertise that adds to our wisdom to exist.

I encourage you to be aware of the situations that arise in your life that make you move from your comfort zone. You may want to log these situations and take note of what changes you think you need to make. I've mentioned (in chapter 5) how to create a manifesto; this would then be the opportunity to create yours, and turn it into your agreement. This is an extraordinary opportunity for growth in every form.

Human beings are infinite travelers, eternal apprentices, inexhaustible adventurers, and pursuers of the inherent brightness of our own diamonds.

CONCLUSION

Love is the religion, and the Universe the book.
—Rumi

The importance of accepting and loving ourselves, despite all the challenges in our health, is the key to success. Our four bodies are connected. They have not separated from each other, and for a complete cure, it is necessary to delve into each body, looking for alignment and perfect health.

This book is a sample of the healing process journey to joy that I took through cancer. Although it has been mainly an intuitive journey, I have read and researched a wide variety of philosophers, doctors, cultures, and scientists—all people from different backgrounds and belief systems. I believe that the bottom line in everything I've done on my journey is related to finding my essence, my truth, which it isn't anything new. Throughout history, human beings, in the end, search for joy of life, truth, and essence.

Lately, the world has been very chaotic. It seems there is too much noise, fear, anxiety, and negative emotions, in general. Yet that shouldn't define us because that is *not* what we are; it's not our nature. That's why I desire to share this book, written with profound honesty and love, hoping that you, the reader, can gain deep insight into your own essence and be your precious self to add goodness and greatness to yourself, your community, and the world.

By sharing my personal experience through cancer and the way I found the connection to inner wisdom, I hope to give valuable information that will help others along their way with cancer and other health issues.

ACKNOWLEDGMENTS

This book would not exist without the unconditional support from my husband and without the love I have received from my children, who have helped me through these hard times. I honor my mother and my biological father for giving me life. I feel blessed to have an adoptive father (stepfather) who has been an example of honesty and dedication to his work. I am grateful for the education that I learned from my parents and for their support. I'm also grateful for my brothers' presence in my life. Despite our age differences, our closeness of heart is immeasurable. Life has united us, and I feel fortunate for it.

I want to thank Rosa Döring, who introduced me to the world of psychoanalysis from the age of seven years old. Thanks to the fact that she has always been a woman of the avant-garde, she introduced me almost two decades ago to the field of the Family Constellations technique and then to the world of bio-decoding—both such powerful healing techniques. From her, I have learned the unimaginable. Thank you, Rosa.

I want to thank Alejandra Hernandez for introducing me to the fascinating world of ThetaHealing, which, for me, was my lifesaver at a crucial moment in my life. My dear friends and ThetaHealers, with whom I have shared so many tears and so many laughs, thank you!

I also want to thank my childhood companions (*El Chal*) for the complicity that has accompanied us from a very early age to date, as well as my career partners, Zoé, Sandra, Claudia, and Tere, who made a stop in their lives to give me their genuine care and love through my process.

Thanks to my friends in Cancun, with whom I share the complicity of motherhood and who have walked every step of this trip with me—Monica, Alejandra, and Maythé. Thanks to my Montessorian friends who have been supporting me in the distance, especially Ana Paulina, for the trust she has placed in me.

Many thanks to Ana Bosch for coming to the rescue, agreeing to be my personal nurse. We have spent hours in pleasant and reflective conversations. Thank you for accompanying me in moments of pain and tears but also of many laughs.

I am so grateful to my neighbors, who have been an incredible support by taking care of my daughters when I needed to be in the clinic.

My love and gratitude to the Trejo, Lozano, Pederzini, Moran, Alamillo, and Escalante families because in the past twenty-five years, a bond has been created that's difficult to break.

I want to thank my doctors in Houston, Texas—my oncologist and thoracic surgeon—whose names are not necessary to mention. These doctors made me pay attention to my inner voice, which shouted that it was me who had to decide what to do with my healing process. I thank their pessimistic and negative words because instead of making me feel defeated, they forced me to feel strong and brave in the uncertain and dark panorama that they proposed me. Despite their attempts to steal my power, they awakened in me the awareness, the strength, and the determination to take control of my health and make the hard decision to dismiss them from my health team. I understand that they are trained in a system; I know that their knowledge (which I respect) is by the book. For me, however, their book is limited and controlled by the strings of a power-hungry pharmaceutical industry. I do believe in conventional medicine, but anything in the extreme can be dangerous.

Thanks to Dr. Deborah Warner (PhD in nutritional science), owner of Clinic Solutions International. She empowered me with the knowledge to create my own path to wellness and taught me to see myself from the DNA perspective. She saved me from an unnecessary surgery. I am very grateful as well to Dr. Robert Rakowski, DC, CCN, DACBN, DIBAK (chiro-practitioner, kinesiologist, certified clinical nutritionist, certified biological terrain instructor, and clinical director of the Natural Medicine Center in Houston, Texas), and Dr. Tanae Romportl, DC, for their commitment and the kindness with which they have always treated me. Both are, first of all, remarkable human beings; I admire their positivism and love their smiles.

I have no words to thank the universe for having been able to find the light in the storm that led me to find Dr. James Forsythe (Forsythe Cancer Center, Reno, Nevada) and his staff, where I also met Dr. Maged, a loving and caring person. Dr. Forsythe's clinic has a group of compassionate human beings committed to the health and wellness of their patients. Thanks as well to Dr. Bruce Fong (Sierra Integrative Medical Center, also in Reno), whose vision of health is 100 percent holistic and respectful of the body, mind, and spirit.

This challenge would have been much harder than normal without the guidance, experience, and compassion of Connie Solera, the closeness of my companions of IGNITE, and, above all, my amethyst sisters (Joan, Carol, Kathy, and Amanda), who filled my healing process with art, creativity, color, solidarity, complicity, laughter, and—beyond everything—much love. I am eternally grateful for your presence. Cynthia, Kate, Kristiann, and Kelly are also my dear IGNITE sisters, who still add so much to my energy with their colorful energy.

I greatly thank Dr. Joe Dispenza for sharing his passion for life, for guiding me to find the missing link in my healing chain, and for showing me the infinite and vast potential that we all have as humans beings and that we can experience life from unimaginable dimensions of possibilities.

Last but not least, I thank the Creator of all that is for being my beacon and my light in the dark. I am infinitely grateful for the opportunity to rebuild me and for its presence in each of my cells that make the magic and miracle of my existence in the highest way and for guiding me to find my secret recipe for my self-healing.

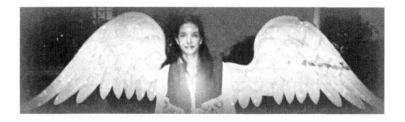

ABOUT THE AUTHOR

Valentina Castro, by nature, likes to serve other individuals. Life, however, prepared a surprise for her. In August 2015, she was diagnosed with Lung Cancer stage IV, a situation that marked a drastic change in her life. She has managed to move forward against the prognosis; at one point in her treatment, she decided to fire her traditional doctors and create her own healing method, following her intuition. This method has helped her and she is now at a point of fullness. Even though the aftermath of cancer remains present, because self-regulation takes time, she successfully overcame cancer's death threat against all prognoses. In the same way, she has helped many people to cope with their health issues (mental and physical) with success.

She studied for a master's of education and children's thinking and has earned a master's degree in clinical psychology and pedagogy and a master's degree in neuropsychology at the Institute of Neurosciences and Mental Health of Barcelona.

Always a very creative person, she began a journey through the world of art therapy and studied Therapeutic Art Education and Development of Self. As a complement to her education, she was trained at Northwestern University in Evanston, Illinois.

She has used art as a therapeutic tool at a domestic-violence shelter and in a school for autistic teenagers. She also has worked for almost twenty years with children, teens, and adults to help them cope with their life problems and has run workshops for groups with different needs.

Valentina was born in Mexico City and moved to Houston, Texas, from 2010 to 2019, where she worked as a therapist for the Epilepsy Foundation in Houston. She also volunteered for a group of Latin women at Unity Church and for a group of low-income immigrant women in the northern Houston. Currently, she's taking a Postgraduate degree in art therapy: "Counseling Expert and

Emotional Regulation Through Art Therapy" at the *Universidad Autónoma de Madrid* (Autonomous University of Madrid) and *Taller Mexicano de Arteterapia, A.C.* (Mexican Art Therapy Workshop School) in Mexico City.

She is a certified ThetaHealer. The ThetaHealing technique is a meditation training technique utilizing a spiritual philosophy for improvement and evolvement of mind, body, and spirit.

THANK YOU

Thanks so much for your interest in this book.

If you have come this far, you must be ready to start the journey and discover the key to your healing process through your four bodies. You're ready to untangle your emotions and find the way out of your labyrinth.

It is my desire to walk you through this challenge, so I created a checklist, a diagnostic assessment to help you find your outlets and your way out of your limiting beliefs that may hold you back on your healing.

www.intuitivearthealing.com.

valcasi@me.com

REFERENCES

- Achterberg, Jeanne. Imagery in Healing. Shambala Publications, Inc. 1995
- Ball, JW, JE Dains, JA Flynn, BS Solomon, and RW Stewart. "Lymphatic System." In *Seidel's Guide to Physical Examination*. Philadelphia, PA: Elsevier Mosby, 2015.
- Braden, Gregg. *La Matriz Divina: Un puente entre el tiempo, el espacio, las creencias y los milagros*. Editorial Sirio, S.A., 2009.
- Champetier de Ribes, Brigitte. *Constelar la Enfermedad desde las comprensiones de Hellinger y Hamer*. Gaia/Grupal, 2013.
- Dispenza, Joe. *You Are the Placebo: Making Your Mind Matter*. United States: Hay House, 2014.
- Gerson, Charlotte. "A Cancer Therapy: Results of Fifty Cases by Dr. Gerson," in *Healing the Gerson Way*, from *Townsend Newsletter*, July 2001.
- Hamer, Dr. Ryke Geerd. *Summary of the New Medicine*. Amici di Dirk, Aug. 1, 2000.
- Hermosillo, Rosa Döring. *Constelaciones, Abrazos y Acuerdos ... Familiares, Otra mirada al pasado para seguir adelante*. Grupo Editorial, 2010.
- Kornfield, Jack. *The Wise Heart: A Guide to the Universal Teachings of Buddhist Psychology*. Bantam Dell, 2008.
- Lipton, Bruce, PhD. *The Biology of Belief: Unleashing the Power of Consciousness, Matter and Miracles*. Hay House Inc., 2008.
- Lowen, Alexander. *El Lenguaje del Cuerpo: Dinámica física de la estructura del character*. Herder Ed, 2010.
- McTaggart, Lynne. *The Power of Eight: Harnessing the Miraculous Energies of a Small Group to Heal Others, Your Life, and the World*. Atria Books, 2017.
- Perez, Mónica Giraldo and Carmen Cecilia Vargas Sierra. *Constelaciones Familiares: Fundamentación sistémica de Bert Hellinger*. Letra Fresca, 2012.

- Rankin, Lissa, MD. *The Fear Cure: Cultivating Courage as Medicine for the Body, Mind, and Soul.* Hay House Inc., 2015.
- Rolf, Eric. *La medicina del Alma.* Madrid, España: Ediciones Gaia, 2003.
- Servan-Scherer, David, MD, PhD. *Anticancer: A Way of Life.* Penguin Group Inc., 2008.
- Stibal, Vianna. *ThetaHealing: Introducing and Extraordinary Energy-Healing Modality.* Hay House, Inc., 2010.
- Trungpa, Chögyam. *The Sanity We Are Born With: a Buddhist Approach to Psychology.* Shambala Publications, Inc., 2005.
- Walker, Morton, DPM. "Liver Detoxification with Coffee Enemas." *Townsend Newsletter,* July 2001.
- *"Sugar Addiction – New Study Validates All Carb Calories Are NOT Created Equal".* JULY 16, 2013 https://universityhealthnews.com/daily/nutrition/sugar-addiction-new-study-validates-all-carb-calories-are-not-created-equal/American Journal of Clinical Nutrition.
- *"Difference between Sympathetic and Parasympathetic Nervous System."* http://www.differencebetween.com/difference-between-sympathetic-and-vs-parasympathetic-nervous-system. 08/15/2018
- *"Natural Killer Cells in Human Cancer: From Biological Functions to Clinical Applications."* https://www.ncbi.nlm.nih.gov/pmc/articles/PMC3085499.
- *"Sugar Addiction."* http://www.childrenshospital.org/centers-and-services/new-balance-foundation-obesity-prevention-center-program/obesity-services.
- "The Importance of Cleansing the Filters of Our Body." https://www.naturopatamasdeu.com/la-importancia-limpiar-los-filtros-de-nuestro-cuerpo.
- "What Is Angiogenesis in Cancer?" https://www.ncbi.nlm.nih.gov/pmc/articles/PMC1993983.

- "What Is BPA?" http://www.mayoclinic.org/healthy-lifestyle/nutrition-and-healthy-eating/expert-answers/bpa/faq-20058331.
- "What Is Psychoneuroimmunology?" http://lapsiconeuroinmunologiauft.blogspot.com.
- "What Is Radiation?" http://www.radiexposure.com.
- "Who Is Christian Fleche?" http://www.christianfleche.com/es/index.php.

Made in the USA
Coppell, TX
15 July 2020